ACTUAL PROBLEMS OF EMERGENCY ABDOMINAL SURGERY

Edited by **Dmitry Victorovich Garbuzenko**

Actual Problems of Emergency Abdominal Surgery

http://dx.doi.org/10.5772/61892
Edited by Dmitry Victorovich Garbuzenko

Contributors

Vincenzo Neri, Julie Reeve, Ianthe Boden, Kate Sullivan, Rebecca Lane, Elroy Weledji, Mehrdad Hosseinpour, Michele Molinari, Ferdane Sapmaz, Sebahat Basyigit, Murat Başaran, Selim Demirci, Alper Yavuz, Çiğdem Hacifazlioğlu, Gökhan Akkurt, Altan Aydın, Hakan Ataş, Marco Massani, Luca Bonariol, Bruno Pauletti, Cesare Ruffolo, Roberta Bonariol, Ezio Caratozzolo, Nicolo' Bassi, Obinna Obinwa, David Cooper, James O'Riordan, Paul Neary, Burhan Hakan Kanat, Buğra Bozan, Seyfi Emir, Selim Sozen, Ilhan Bali, Mehmet Burak Dal, Fatih Erol, Esra Caliskan, Andrei Beliaev, Michael Booth

Published by InTech

Janeza Trdine 9, 51000 Rijeka, Croatia

Publishing Process Manager Andrea Koric

Technical Editor SPi Global

Cover InTech Design team

First published September, 2016

Printed in Croatia

Additional hard copies can be obtained from orders@intechopen.com

Actual Problems of Emergency Abdominal Surgery, Edited by Dmitry Victorovich Garbuzenko

p. cm.

Print ISBN 978-953-51-2646-1
Online ISBN 978-953-51-2647-8

For EU product safety concerns:
IN TECH d.o.o., Prolaz Marije Krucifikse Kozulić 3, 51000 Rijeka, Croatia,
info@intechopen.com or visit our website at intechopen.com.

Meet the editor

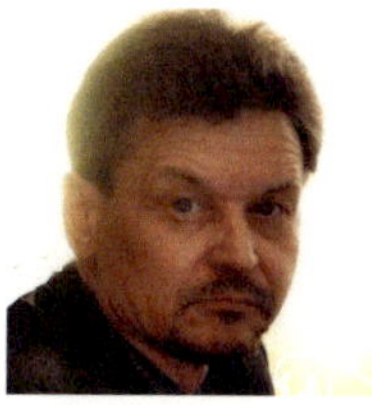

Prof. Dmitry Victorovich Garbuzenko, MD, PhD, was born in 1962 in Russia. In 1985, he graduated from the Chelyabinsk State Medical Academy. From 1985 to 1990, he was a post-graduate student in Department of Hospital Surgery, ChSMA. Since 1990, D.V. Garbuzenko has been working in the South Ural State Medical University as professor in Department of Faculty Surgery. He is surgeon of the highest category. All of his practical activity was devoted to emergency abdominal surgery. Prof. Garbuzenko is a member of the Russian Society of Surgeons and the International Association of Surgeons-Hepatologists. He has authored more than 130 publications, 3 inventions, and 2 monographs ("Gastroesophageal variceal hemorrhage in cirrhotic patients: pathogenesis, prophylactic, treatment" and "Selected lectures in emergency abdominal surgery"). The editor of the book "Portal Hypertension: Causes and Complications" in Rijeka Croatia from InTech, 2012.

Contents

Preface

Proper organization and quality of medical care in emergency surgical diseases depend largely on the availability of knowledgeable and highly trained professionals. Good literature plays an important role in their preparation.

The book "Actual Problems of Emergency Abdominal Surgery" was written by an international team of authors with extensive practical experience. It contains literature reviews describing some of the diseases and pathological conditions that occur in emergency surgical practice. The book consists of three sections devoted to abdominal surgery, abdominal trauma, and pediatric surgery.

Section "Abdominal Surgery" includes seven chapters. In them, the authors describe the problems associated with the diagnosis and treatment of acute appendicitis and acute intestinal obstruction, examine the risk factors for complications of laparoscopic cholecystectomy, emphasize the importance of timely diagnosis of rectosigmoid perforation, talk about the principles of management of patients with foreign bodies of the gastrointestinal tract, raise the question of the differential diagnosis of abdominal pain, and indicate the role of physiotherapy in the postoperative management of patients.

Acute appendicitis is one of the most common diseases in emergency abdominal surgery. Timely diagnosis is the key to its successful treatment. However, in some cases, there are difficulties with the identification of acute appendicitis, particularly in women of childbearing age, pregnant women, infants, and elderly patients. They may delay surgery and contribute to the increase of complications and mortality.

Acute intestinal obstruction is one of the main reasons for admission of patients to the surgical hospitals. Among all patients with mechanical intestinal obstruction, acute small bowel obstruction is the most common. It is characterized by severe clinical course and poor prognosis. The primary cause of acute large bowel obstruction is colorectal cancer. In severe cases, it is accompanied by a high level of mortality and the frequent development of postoperative complications. Strangulation is the most dangerous type of intestinal obstruction requiring emergency surgery.

In the structure of acute surgical diseases, acute cholecystitis takes second place after acute appendicitis. Higher quality of its treatment became possible owing to the widespread introduction of minimally invasive surgical technology into clinical practice. Nevertheless, in some cases, there are situations that require the conversion of laparoscopic cholecystectomy to open surgery. Risk stratification for complications associated with laparoscopic cholecystectomy is an actual problem of biliary surgery.

Rectosigmoid perforation is a rare complication in emergency surgery. It is necessary to remember the causes that contribute to its development and to be able to diagnose it in a timely manner.

In some cases, a doctor may encounter certain difficulties in managing patients with foreign bodies in the gastrointestinal tract. A competent individual approach in these cases allows avoiding related complications.

Currently, no one doubts that one of the critical circumstances that reduces mortality in acute surgical diseases of the abdomen is their timely diagnosis in the prehospital phase. Unfortunately, this does not always happen in practice, sometimes due to wrong interpretation of abdominal pain. Ability to understand their reason is exceedingly important for a general practitioner.

There are few publications about the role of physiotherapy after emergency surgery. Nevertheless, the outcome of the disease may depend on the quality of postoperative management of patients.

Section "Abdominal Trauma" includes three chapters devoted to injuries of the liver and intra- and extrahepatic biliary tract and the principles of management of patients according to the program "Damage Control".

Liver injury is the most severe abdominal trauma, which is difficult to diagnose and treat. In recent years, the problem of assisting in liver trauma is becoming increasingly important owing to the increase in transport and industrial accidents, the criminalization of society, and military conflicts. Timely diagnosis, selection of the optimal treatment strategy, and the use of modern technology in liver trauma will reduce associated morbidity and mortality.

One of the dangerous complications of liver trauma is a bile peritonitis, which results in, as a rule, injuries of the intra- and extrahepatic biliary tract. Their timely diagnosis allows avoiding this serious complication. The nature of surgery depends on the pathology identified during the examination of the abdominal cavity.

The program "Damage Control" provides an implementation of the programmed multistage surgical treatment of victims admitted to the hospital in critical condition. Its introduction into practice of the leading specialized centers for the treatment of concomitant injuries can reduce mortality in the most difficult group of victims in critical condition.

Section "Pediatric Surgery" includes two chapters, one of which tells about the most frequent causes of acute abdomen in children, and the other is devoted to providing anesthesia in emergency surgery in newborns. It is clear that emergency pediatric surgery has its own characteristics, knowledge of which is essential for a general surgeon.

Thus, the problems described are relevant for emergency abdominal surgery. We hope that the materials of the book will be of interest to anyone who considers it his or her specialty.

Professor Dmitry Victorovich Garbuzenko
Department of Faculty Surgery,
South Ural State Medical University,
Chelyabinsk, Russia

Section 1

Abdominal Surgery

Chapter 1

The Dilemma of Acute Appendicitis

Elroy Patrick Weledji

Additional information is available at the end of the chapter

http://dx.doi.org/10.5772/63097

Abstract

Acute appendicitis is one of a relatively dwindling number of conditions in which a decision to operate may be based solely on clinical findings. Regular re-assessment of patients and making use of the investigative options available will meet the standard of care expected by patients with acute abdominal pain. In this article, the greater importance of history and examination over investigations in the early diagnosis of acute appendicitis is emphasized. The ability to identify the presence of peritoneal inflammation probably has the greatest influence on the final surgical decision.

Keywords: acute appendicitis, assessment, differential diagnosis, management, outcome

1. Introduction

Acute appendicitis is the most common cause of the acute abdomen requiring surgery with a life-time risk of ~7%, which is maximal in childhood and declines steadily with age as the lymphoid tissue and vascularity atrophy [1, 2]. Surgery for the acute abdomen caused by appendicitis only evolved when the mortality associated with perforated appendicitis was found to be high. Conservative treatment with later drainage of any abscess had been the standard and diffuse peritonitis was usually fatal. Although only few patients progressed to the potentially lethal complications, early surgery for all patients with suspected appendicitis became the definitive method of preventing severe peritoneal sepsis [2–4]. Although a study demonstrated that simple appendicitis may be treated with antibiotics only, there is a risk of recurrent attacks [4]. Recent advances in interventional radiological techniques for peritonitis have significantly reduced the morbidity and mortality of physiologically severe complicated abdominal infection [5]. However, when there is clinical suspicion of the acute abdomen, the best policy is early surgery if diagnostic tools are not readily available. The mortality of perforated viscus increases with delay in diagnosis and management, and it is greatest in the elderly and those ill from intercurrent disease with a poor performance status (ASA score) [2, 6–9].

2. Natural history

The natural history of acute appendicitis left untreated is that it will either resolve spontaneously by host defenses or progress to a fatal suppurative necrosis (gangrene) with perforation. The appendicular artery is a single end artery closely applied to the wall distally, and secondary thrombosis is common giving rise to gangrene which explains the short progressive history (3–5 days) of appendicitis and the poorer prognosis with the artherosclerosis of the aged. The classical presentation is referred, dull, poorly localized, colicky periumbilical pain (visceral) from the luminal obstruction (mid-gut origin) for 12–24 hours that shifts and localizes to the right iliac fossa as peritoneal irritation by the inflamed appendix occurs (somatic pain). There is nausea but vomiting more than twice is rare. A low grade pyrexia and constipation is usual [2]. An alternative outcome is that the appendix becomes surrounded by a mass of omentum or adjacent viscera which walls off the inflammatory process and prevents inflammation spreading to the abdominal cavity yet resolution of the condition is delayed (appendix mass). Such a patient usually presents with a longer history (a week or more) of right lower quadrant abdominal pain, appears systemically well and has a tender palpable mass in the right iliac fossa. Conservative management risks a 30% recurrence of acute inflammation [3, 8, 10]. Subacute obstruction may occur in the elderly and the appendix mass may be confused with a caecal carcinoma, Crohn's disease, tuberculosis or an ovarian tumour. However, a mass is often detected only after the patient has been anaesthesized and paralysed. Thus, the differentiation of a phlegmonous mass from an abscess is not a practical problem because surgery is the correct management for both. Such a policy renders any debate on interval appendicectomy redundant [3]. The operation which may be an appendicectomy, an ileocaecal resection or a hemicolectomy if indicated during the first admission is expeditious and safe, provided steps are taken to minimize postoperative sepsis [2, 3, 11]. The serious consequences of missing a carcinoma in the elderly patient are abolished [3].

3. Clinical assessment

Just as appendicitis should be considered in any patient with abdominal pain, virtually every other abdominal emergency can be considered in the differential diagnosis of suspected appendicitis. Clues to the differential diagnosis include recent sore throat (mesenteric adenitis), previous episode (Crohn's disease), weight loss (Crohn's disease, caecal carcinoma), dyspepsia (cholecystitis, perforated ulcer), arthralgia (*Yersinia enterocolitica*, Crohn's disease), vaginal discharge (salpingitis), mid-menstrual cycle (ruptured follicular cyst), frequency (urinary tract infection), preserved appetite (non-specific, or gynaecological) and

Asian origin (ileocaecal tuberculosis) [3]. In acute appendicitis the point of maximum tenderness (*McBurney's point*) usually lies one-third along a line from the anterior superior iliac spine to the umbilicus which denotes the surface anatomy of the appendix. This is associated with guarding of the inflamed area from being prodded further [2, 12, 13]. Although not of diagnostic value as being non-specific, pressure in the left iliac fossa produces pain in the right iliac fossa (*Rovsing's sign*) [14]. Occasionally, patients with appendicitis have signs of widespread peritonitis, which obscure the area of maximal tenderness. Re-examination, after resuscitation and adequate analgesia, permits more reliable localization of signs [2, 3, 13, 14]. The appendix can occasionally be in different positions within the abdomen and can lead to the pain localizing in more unusual places, which may lead to a delay in diagnosis. A retrocaecal appendix can give rise to tenderness in the right upper quadrant, whereas a pelvic appendix may be associated with central abdominal discomfort. Passive extension or hyperextension of the hip increases the abdominal pain because of an inflamed appendix lying on the psoas muscle (*Psoas stretch test*). The *obturator sign* is positive when passive internal rotation of the hip aggravates the pain of an inflamed appendix lying on the obturator internus, but, an ovarian pathology may do same [2, 3, 15]. Left-sided appendicitis is a rare and atypical presentation associated with congenital midgut malrotation, situs inversus or an abnormally long appendix [16]. The apex beat of the heart on the right side will betray the diagnosis if there is associated dextrocardia. When rebound tenderness is detected in the lower abdomen, further examination by rectal examination has been shown to provide no new information. Rectal examination is reserved for those patients without rebound tenderness or where specific pelvic disease needs to be excluded. It is of little value in the diagnosis of acute appendicitis even when the organ lies in the pelvis [17]. The demonstration and interpretation of these physical signs are skills that fade without practice. The age, sex and personality of the patient are important modifiers of clinical signs; the most typical cases occur in older children (5–15 years) of either sex and in young males with poor dietary fibre being a risk factor. In other individuals, the features are more obscure, and the potential for alternative pathology is greater [2, 3]. It is, however, not possible to practice fully the ideal management of early diagnosis and surgery for the acute abdomen, thus reducing morbidity and mortality to zero, because patients and the disease are variable. Nevertheless, because infection, inadequate tissue perfusion and a persistent inflammatory state are the most important risk factors for development of multiple organ failure, it seems logical that initial therapeutic efforts should be directed at their early treatment or prevention (early goal-directed therapy). The risk of portal pyaemia from septic emboli is also decreased [10]. It is important to recognize the features of the acute abdomen which would indicate the need for resuscitation in the high dependency or intensive care unit [11]. The attitude of the patient with advanced peritonitis is best described by Hippocrates (460–370 B.C.) as one with a 'sharp nose, hollow eyes, collapsed temples, the ears cold' now known as the *Hippocratic facies*. The patient is usually ill and clammy, hypotensive with a rapid thready pulse. The patient will lie perfectly still to minimize discomfort, the abdomen held totally rigid as the patient takes rapid shallow breaths using chest movements only [18].

4. Any role for the Alvarado score?

The Alvarado score was designed more than two decades ago as a diagnostic score using the clinical features of acute appendicitis for subsequent clinical management but the appropriateness for its routine clinical use is still unclear (**Table 1**) [19]. A recent meta-analysis showed its positive role in 'ruling out' appendicitis but not in 'ruling in' the diagnosis without surgical assessment and further diagnostic testing. It is inconsistent in children and over-predicts the probability of acute appendicitis in women [20]. Alvarado scoring may be valuable in low-resource or primary care centres where imaging is not an option.

Symptoms	Migration	1
	Anorexia-acetone	1
	Nausea-vomiting	1
Signs	Tenderness in right lower quadrant	2
	Rebound pain	1
	Elevation of temperature	1
Laboratory	Leukocytosis	2
	Shift to the left	1
Total score		10

A score of 5 or 6 is compatible with the diagnosis of acute appendicitis. A score of 7 or 8 indicates a probable appendicitis, and a score of 9 or 10 indicates a very probable appendicitis.

Table 1. Mnemonic for the diagnostic score of acute appendicitis.

4.1. Any role for special investigations in appendicitis?

There are no special investigations to confirm appendicitis. As no test is accurate, the diagnosis has to rely on clinical symptoms and signs [2, 3, 18]. Tests should serve as adjuncts to clinical diagnosis and may help to exclude alternative diagnoses especially in the female or the elderly [3]. A white cell count is usually elevated but a normal white cell count does not exclude appendicitis [19, 20]. The appendicolith, a radio-opaque concretion located within the appendix, which is deemed to be the most specific finding of appendicitis on plain radiographs, is visualized in only 5–15% of patients with appendicitis [21]. Ultrasonography in expert hands is perhaps the most useful investigation [2, 3, 21]. Although computed tomography (CT) scan is superior to ultrasound (US) scan, the risk of radiation-induced malignancy renders it not of particular use in paediatric patients [21]. Laparoscopy is essentially an operation rather than an investigation. However, the continuing development of ultrasound techniques and laparoscopic surgery have both prompted the view that the proportion of normal appendices removed (20%) is unacceptably high [22]. Although it is clearly advantageous to spare patients from unnecessary surgery, the morbidity and mortality of failing to diagnose appendicitis until perforation has occurred is greater than that associated with removal of normal appendix [2, 3].

4.2. If diagnostic tools not readily available

The best policy is early surgery when there is clinical suspicion of acute appendicitis. If the appendix is macroscopically normal, the terminal 60 cm of ileum must be delivered to exclude a Meckel's diverticulum, terminal ileitis and mesenteric adenitis. If the base of the appendix and caecum are healthy, the appendix must be removed when ileitis is present [2, 3]. Biopsy and culture of inflamed nodes aids a diagnosis of *Yersinia* infection. The right ovary and tube must be visualized. Extension of the incision, a head down tilt and adequate retraction may be required. Occasionally, fluid leaking from a perforated peptic ulcer down the right paracolic gutter produces clinical findings resembling those of acute appendicitis. A classical appendicectomy incision would reveal bile-staining free peritoneal fluid and a second upper abdominal incision is usually required. Purulent fluid tracking down the right paracolic gutter may also suggest acute cholecystitis. If clinical diagnosis is equivocal despite investigations, it is best to begin with a low midline incision which could be extended if there is evidence of a perforated peptic ulcer [2, 23].

5. The diagnostic dilemma

5.1. The young woman

It is not surprising that women have the highest appendicectomy rate with 30% revealing normal appendices [16, 24]. In young women, various gynaecological conditions are present with lower abdominal pain, and the history gives important clues. Vaginal discharge, a longer history (often more than 72 hours) and absence of gastrointestinal upset raise the possibility of pelvic inflammatory disease. A bilateral, low distribution of pain aggravated by cervical movement support the diagnosis [24]. Abrupt onset of pain suggests rupture of a follicle, cyst or ectopic gestation [25]. The condition of *Curtis-Fitz-Hugh syndrome* when transperitoneal spread of pelvic inflammatory disease produces pain in right upper quadrant due to perihepatic adhesions is now well recognized, and care must be taken to distinguish this from acute biliary conditions [25]. Early recognition with diagnostic laparoscopy and appropriate treatment of pelvic inflammatory disease may help to avoid potentially serious longer term sequelae and must be encouraged. Many studies have now demonstrated that laparoscopy significantly improves surgical decision-making in patients with acute abdominal pain especially in the young woman [16, 22, 24].

5.2. Chronic appendicitis or 'the grumbling appendix'

Patients with true relapsing or chronic appendicitis are rare, and often it is difficult to diagnose as the symptoms may be atypical and short-lived. In genuine cases, the macroscopic appearance of the appendix is abnormal, and thus the diagnosis is best established by laparoscopy, following which the appendix can be removed [22]. Minor frequent episodes of right iliac fossa pain 'the grumbling appendix' can be caused by thread worms in the appendix or by some conditions other than the appendix. Chronic pain with evidence of organic disease (weight loss, elevated erythrocyte sedimentation rate (ESR)) is usually due to Crohn's disease at any age, caecal carcinoma in the elderly or lymphoma or tuberculosis in endemic areas [2, 22, 23]. Pain without signs or abnormal investigations is likely to be due to irritable bowel syndrome, but small bowel studies are still warranted if pain persists, to exclude more unusual causes [3].

5.3. The pregnant woman

Acute appendicitis is the most common general surgical problem encountered during pregnancy confirmed in 1:800 to 1:1500 pregnancies [26]. Difficulty in diagnosis, reluctance to operate a pregnant women and avoidable delay account for the high risks of appendicitis in pregnancy. In pregnancy, the enlarging uterus progressively displaces the appendix up into the right hypochondrium. Delay is so harmful to mother and unborn child that provided urinary tract infection has been excluded, one should operate early. Maternal and fetal deaths do not result from appendicectomy but from peritonitis following perforation. The risk of maternal mortality increases as pregnancy progresses [27].

5.4. The elderly and the infant

Appendicitis has a more rapid course in the elderly as artherosclerosis, gangrene and perforation are common. Its atypical presentation adds to the delay in diagnosis [9]. A diagnosis of carcinoma of the caecum or lymphoma, which has obstructed the appendix, must be considered and excluded by CT scan [3]. Diagnosis of acute appendicitis may be difficult in infants. Delay in diagnosis is common because the classical signs and symptoms may be absent or unobtainable, and perforation is common as host defenses including the omentum are not fully developed. The development of fever associated with any abdominal tenderness should always raise the suspicion of acute appendicitis [2, 21]. 'Active observation' is safe and effective in early appendicitis and in patients where the diagnosis is in doubt. It permits differentiation between patients with persistent or progressive signs requiring surgery and those with non-specific pain or alternative pathology [3, 28]. Deliberate delay allows time for the results of appropriate investigations to be reviewed, and it is extremely rare for such an appendix to rupture during observation and the diagnosis will usually become apparent within 12–24 hours [29].

5.5. The AIDS patient

Abdominal pain is common in patients with AIDS, but less than 1% of patients with AIDS will need an emergency laparotomy [30]. The commonest disease processes, *cytomegalovirus* (CMV) colitis, B-cell lymphoma, acute appendicitis (CMV-associated) and atypical mycobacterial infection are quite different from those in the non-HIV population. These patients are difficult to manage as it is often unclear whether they need an immediate laparotomy. It is crucial to have close liaison between AIDS physicians and AIDS surgeons to exclude pre-terminal cases and keep down negative laparotomies to acceptable rate. Appendicectomy and colectomy are the commonest abdominal operations in AIDS patients [31]. Being an extranodal lymphoid organ appendicitis could be the only initial indication of a lymphoma or lymphadenopathy from *Myocobacterium avium-intracellulare* obstructing the appendiceal ostium. Thus appendicectomy specimens should routinely be examined histologically [32]. With careful patient selection, emergency laparotomy confers worthwhile palliation [30, 31, 33]. However, some patients (and their families) refuse surgery in desperate situations (such as bowel perforation) as they want an end to the suffering [31, 33].

6. Conclusions

A precise history of the acute abdomen may indicate the pathology, and physical examination may indicate where the pathology is. However, the ability to identify the presence of peritoneal inflammation probably has the greatest influence on the final surgical decision. The best policy is early surgery when there is clinical suspicion of the acute abdomen if diagnostic tools are not readily available, but 'active observation' is effective and safe in early appendicitis. Regular re-assessment of patients and making use of the investigative options available will meet the standard of care expected by patients with acute abdominal pain.

Conflict of interest: The author declares that there is no conflict of interest.

Contributorship: E.P. Weledji is the sole author of this article.

Funding acknowledgement: This research received no specific grant from any funding agency in the public, commercial or not-for-profit sectors.

Author details

Elroy Patrick Weledji

Address all correspondence to: elroypat@yahoo.co.uk

Department of Surgery, Faculty of Health Sciences, University of Buea, Cameroon, West Africa

References

[1] Ergul E. Importance of family history and genetics for the prediction of acute appendicitis. Internet J Surg 2007, 10:2.

[2] Krukowski ZH, O'Kelly TJ. Appendicitis. Surgery 1997, 15:76–81.

[3] Bailey I, Tate JJT. Acute conditions of the small bowel and appendix (including perforated peptic ulcer) pp:187–212. In: Patterson-Brown S (ed), Emergency surgery and critical care. A companion to Specialist Surgical Practice 1997 WB Saunders Company ltd : 24-28 Oval Road London NW1 7DX.

[4] Fitzmaurice GJ, McWilliams B, Hurreiz H, Epanomertakis E. Antibiotics versus appendectomy in the management of acute appendicitis: a review of the current evidence. Can J Surg 2011, 54(5):307–314.

[5] Solomon J, Mazuski J. Intraabdominal sepsis: newer interventional and antimicrobial therapies. Infect Dis Clin N Am 2009, 23: 593–608.

[6] Marshall JC, Maier RV, Jimerz M et al. Source control in the management of severe sepsis and septic shock: an evidence-based review. Crit Care Med 2004, 32:5513–5526.

[7] River SE, Nguyen B, Haystd S, et al. Early goal-directed therapy in the treatment of severe sepsis and septic shock. N Eng J Med 2001, 345:1368–1377.

[8] Baigrie RJ, Dehn TCB, Fowler SM, Dunn DC. Analysis of 8651 appendicectomies in England and Wales during 1992. Br J Surg 1995, 82:933.

[9] Hardy K, Ackermann C, Hewitt J. The acute abdomen in the older person. Scott Med J February 2013, 58:41–45.

[10] Marik PE. Surviving sepsis: going beyond the guidelines. Ann Intensive Care 2011; 1(1): 17.

[11] Weledji EP, Ngowe NM. The challenge of intraabdominal sepsis. Int J Surg 2013, 11(4): 290–295.

[12] Gallegos N, Hobsley N. Abdominal pain: parietal or visceral. J R Soc Med 1992, 85:379.

[13] Bennett DH, Tambeur LJMT, Campbell WB. Use of coughing test to diagnose peritonitis. Br Med J 1994, 308:1336–1337.

[14] Smith PH. The diagnosis of appenicitis. Postgrad Med Journ 1965, 41:2–5.

[15] Stevens L, Kenney A. Emergencies in Obstetrics and Gynaecology. Oxford University Press, Oxford, 1994.

[16] Yang CY, Lin HY, Lin HL, Lin JN. Left-sided acute appendicitis: a pitfall in the emergency department. J Emerg Med 2012, 43(6):980–982.

[17] Dixon JM, Elton R. Rectal examination in patients with pain in the right lower quadrant of the abdomen. Br Med J 1991, 302:386–388.

[18] Bailey H, Bishop WJ. The Hippocratic facies. In: Notable names in Medicine and Surgery 3rd Edn 1959. Published by H.K. Lewis & Co. Ltd. London 1959.

[19] Alvarado A. A practical score for the early diagnosis of acute appendicitis. Ann Emerg Med 1986, 15(5):557–564.

[20] Ohle R, O'Reilly F, O'Brien KK, Fahey T, Dimitrov BD. The Alvarado score for predicting acute appendicitis: a systematic review. BMC Med 2011, 9:139.

[21] Brennan GDG. Paediatric appendicitis: pathophysiology and appropriate use of diagnosing imaging. Can J Emerg Med 2006, 8(6):425–432.

[22] Paterson-Brown S, Eckersley JRT. Laparoscopy as an adjunct to decision-making in the acute abdomen. Br J Surg 1986, 73:1022–1024.

[23] Paterson-Brown S. Diagnosis and investigation in the acute abdomen. In: Paterson-Brown S (ed), Emergency Surgery and Critical Care. A Companion to Specialist Surgical Practice. W.B.Saunders, 1997.

[24] Pearce JM. Pelvic inflammatory disease. Br Med J 1990, 300:1090–1091.

[25] Gatt D, Heafield T, Jantet G. Curtis–Fitz-Hugh syndrome: the new mimicking disease. Ann R Coll Surg Eng 1986, 68:271–274.

[26] Andersen B, Nielsen TF. Appendicitis in pregnancy: diagnosis, management and complications. Acta Obstet Gynecol Scand 1999, 78:758.

[27] Mourad J, Elliott JP, Erickson L, Lisboa L. Appendicitis in pregnancy: new information that contradicts long-held clinical beliefs. Am J Obstet Gynecol 2000, 182:1027.

[28] Thompson HJ, Jones PF. Acute observation in acute abdominal pain. Am J Surg 1986, 132:522–555.

[29] Moss JG, Barrie Jl, Gunn AA. Delay in surgery for acute appendicitis. J R Coll Surg Edinb 1985, 30:290–293.

[30] Dua RS, Wajed SA, Winsler MC. Impact of HIV and AIDS on surgical practice. Ann R Coll Surg Engl 2007, 89:354–358.

[31] Smit S. Guidelines for surgery in the HIV patients (Continuous Medical Education (CME): August 2010, 28, No 8.

[32] Weledji EP, Ngowe MN, Abba JS. Burkitt's lymphoma masquerading as acute appendicitis–two case reports and review of the literature. World J Surg Oncol 2014, 12:187.

[33] Weledji EP, Nsagha D, Chichom AM, Enoworock G. Gastrointestinal surgery and the acquired immune deficiency syndrome. Ann Med Surg (Lond) 2015, 4(1):36–40.

Chapter 2

Management of Intestinal Obstruction

Vincenzo Neri

Additional information is available at the end of the chapter

http://dx.doi.org/10.5772/63156

Abstract

Objective: Intestinal obstruction is a blockage of the intestinal content through bowel. The block must be complete and permanent. Obstruction may be mechanical, simple or strangulated, and paralytic. The purpose of this chapter is to clarify, also evaluating our surgical experience, the steps to diagnose and the ways to treat intestinal obstructions.

Methods: In the period 2011–2015, we have treated 52 patients with the clinical presentation of intestinal obstruction. Acute mechanical small bowel obstructions were the most frequent (71.2%), whereas acute large bowel obstructions were the less frequent (28.8%). Some steps in the physical examination and plain radiography are as follows:

- Preliminary diagnosis: simple versus strangulated obstruction.
- First-step diagnosis: mechanical or paralytic obstruction.
- Second-step diagnosis (define the level of obstruction).
- Third-step diagnosis: kind of obstacle.

Results: In our experience, all complete intestinal obstructions have been treated with urgent surgery. Various types of surgical procedures have been employed based on intraoperative pathological findings

Conclusion: Surgical emergency is the first choice of treatment in strangulation obstruction and in simple (complete) mechanical obstruction of small and large bowel. Generally, paralytic ileus can be resolved with the treatment that caused it. Intestinal pseudo-obstruction is a syndrome characterized by a complete dilatation generally of large bowel without mechanical obstacle. The chronic pseudo-obstruction can be idiopathic or secondary to systemic disease.

Keywords: intestinal management, obstruction, pathophysiology, strangulation, intestinal pseudo-obstruction

1. Introduction

Intestinal obstruction is a syndrome characterized by a blockage of the intestinal content, gas and liquid, through small or large bowel. The block must be complete and permanent.

There are several data that can diversify the intestinal obstruction syndrome. First, the etiology based on a large number of factors that allow the subdivision into mechanical and functional/ paralytic obstruction.

The other feature characterizes the syndrome: the seat of the obstruction along the bowel— upper small gut, distal small gut, and large bowel.

Finally, the cause of obstruction can involve the vascular supply of an intestinal segment, giving rise to strangulation obstruction that should be differentiated from simple obstruction.

The syndrome of intestinal obstruction with these various etiopathological and clinical features develops the same, overlappable, and pathophysiological alterations.

2. Etiology

Bowel obstruction can be caused by several factors.

The causes of mechanical obstruction can be divided into causes within the bowel lumen, causes in the intestinal wall, and extrinsic causes.

The causes within the bowel are infrequent. They can be due to large gallstones passed into the intestinal lumen by spontaneous bilio-digestive fistulas, most frequently cholecystoduodenal fistulas, very rarely phito-thricobezoar, masses of parasites, food bolus, concretions of barium following barium enema X-ray investigation or X-ray studies with opaque medium.

It is useful to point out that the fecaloma, fecal impaction in the rectal ampulla, based on the damage of the autonomic nervous system in the colorectal wall, can cause chronic alteration of intestinal transit with incomplete obstruction without the pathophysiological alterations of acute gut obstruction.

The causes in the gut wall include the neoplasms of small and large bowel, the congenital atresias, the stenosis due to chronic inflammatory disease (Crohn disease, diverticulitis, etc.), and postanastomotic or posttraumatic structures.

The extrinsic causes include a very large range of pathological conditions: compression by external masses, adhesions, bands, strangulated external or internal hernias, volvulus, and intussusception [1]. In the clinical practice, it should be valuable to distinguish between acute and chronic obstructions. Nevertheless to define both clinical pictures with accuracy is very useful. The acute intestinal obstruction, simple or strangulated forms, is characterized by complete and permanent blockage and consequently the acute pathophysiological syndrome of obstruction may develop with all clinical, laboratory, and instrumental features: bowel dilatation, disturbances of fluids and electrolytes balance, congestion, and ischemic parietal damage, etc.

On the contrary, in the chronic obstruction, the blockage of gut transit is incomplete and the syndrome cannot develop completely and is characterized only by constipation.

3. Classification of intestinal obstruction

Intestinal obstruction may be mechanical or paralytic. Mechanical obstruction can be due to intraluminal, intrinsic to the intestinal wall and extrinsic.

Paralytic ileus due to reduction or the absence of peristalsis can be caused by peritoneal phlogosis, infection, abdominal surgery, pelvic surgery, and some medications such as antidepressant, pain medications, muscle and nerve disorders, and retroperitoneal hemorrhage.

The majority of patients have simple obstruction. On the contrary, there is also strangulation obstruction, usually due to complicated external hernia (abdominal wall) or internal (by congenital defects or postoperative adhesions): in these patients the vascular supply to a strangulated intestinal segment is compromised and consequently intestinal infarction. Strangulation obstruction leads to an increased risk of morbidity and mortality.

In the mechanical occlusion with strangulation, the vascular (arterial and venous) occlusion leads to bowel ischemia and necrosis. The evolution of strangulated bowel is the perforation and peritonitis. The occlusive syndrome becomes worse due to strangulation.

Intestinal pseudo-obstruction is a syndrome characterized by a complete dilatation generally of large bowel without mechanical obstacle. The intestinal pseudo-obstruction can affect small or large bowel and it may be possible to differentiate the syndromes with acute or chronic onset and evolution.

The chronic pseudo-obstruction can be idiopathic or secondary to systemic disease.

4. Epidemiology

The examination of homogeneous clinical cases of a single center allows us to clarify the epidemiological features.

In the period 2011–2015, 52 patients have been admitted in our service with the clinical presentation of intestinal obstruction.

Demographic data are as follows: 52 patients, 26 males, 26 females, and mean age 67 years (range 27–86 years).

Acute mechanical small bowel obstruction was the most frequent (71.2%) with various pathologies: adhesion -relate obstructions, small bowel volvulus, gallstones ileus, malignancies, abdominal wall hernias, internal hernias, carcinomatosis, and ileocecocolic intussusception (**Figure 1**).

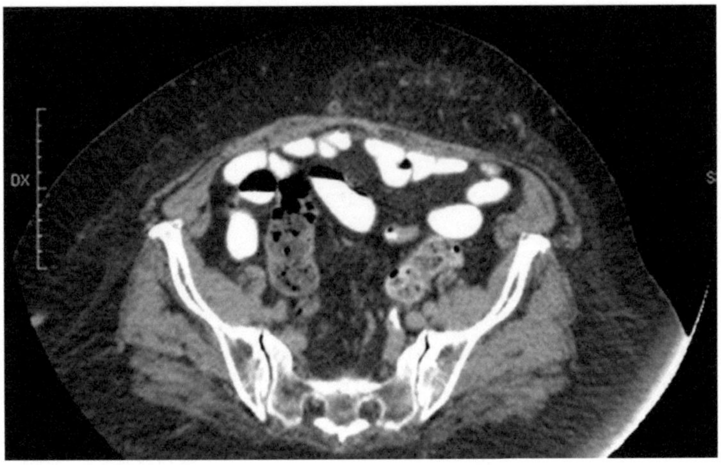

Figure 1. CT scan: ileocecocolic intussusceptions.

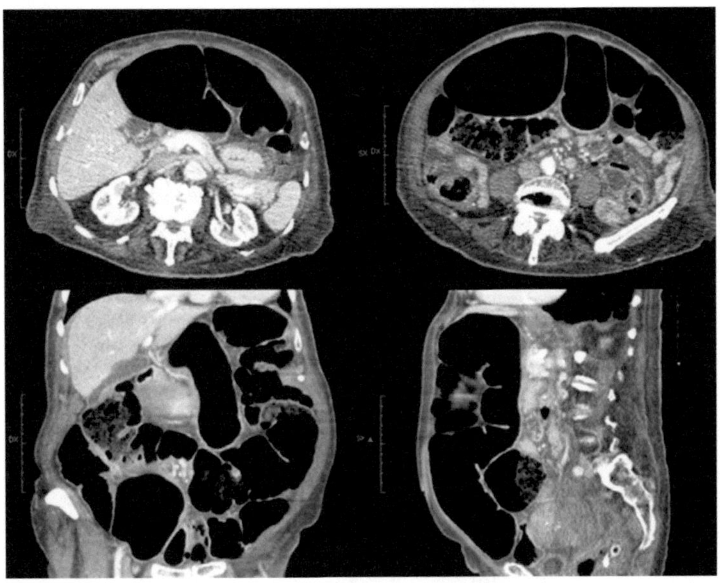

Figure 2. CT scan: sigmoid volvulus.

The less frequent in our experience were acute large bowel obstructions (28.8%). The more common pathologies were colon and rectal cancer, sigmoid volvulus (**Figure 2**). We have observed and treated only one patient with acute colonic pseudo-obstruction (Ogilvie's syndrome) (**Table 1**).

	n	%
Adhesions	22	42.3
Small bowel volvulus	4	7.7
Sigmoid volvulus	1	1.9
Right colon cancer	3	5.8
Left colon cancer	5	9.6
Rectal cancer	5	9.6
Ogilvie's syndrome	1	1.9
Gallstones ileus	2	3.8
Carcinomatosis	1	1.9
Strangulated incisional hernia	3	5.8
Strangulated groin hernia	2	3.8
Strangulated umbilical hernia	1	1.9
Internal hernia	1	1.9
Ileocecocolic intussusception	1	1.9
Total	52	

Table 1. Fifty-two acute intestinal obstructions: pathologies.

	n	%
Adhesiolysis	18	34.6%
Small bowel resection	6	11.5
Right hemicolectomy	4	7.7
Left hemicolectomy	5	9.6
Intestinal derotation	4	7.7
Cecostomy	2	3.8
Enterotomy and gallstone removal	2	3.8
Anterior rectum resection	4	7.7
Total colectomy	1	1.9
Prosthetic mesh repair incisional hernia	3	5.8
Umbilical hernia repair	1	1.9
Prosthetic mesh repair groin hernia	2	3.8
	52	

Table 2. Fifty-two acute intestinal obstructions: surgical interventions.

In our experience, all intestinal obstructions have been treated with urgent surgery. Various types of surgical procedures have been employed based on intraoperative pathological findings. They should be useful to underline that the choice of the urgent treatment allowed the resolution of majority of adhesion-related obstructions and small bowel volvulus with the surgical procedure of adhesiolysis and intestinal derotation (42.3%). The intestinal resection has been performed in six cases (11.5%). Ogilvie's syndrome required cecostomy; colorectal malignancies have been treated with primary tumors resection and delayed intestinal anastomosis. Our surgical interventions are reported in **Table 2**.

5. Pathophysiology of simple intestinal obstruction

In simple obstruction, important and progressive alterations take place and develop in the gut above the obstruction. Accumulation of gas and liquids with progressive distension in intestinal segments upstream the obstruction and the blockage of content progress change the bacteriological content. Also there are damages of blood circulation in the distended bowel wall. The accumulation of fluid and electrolytes in the obstructed gut and their loss in the general circulation take an important place in the pathophysiology of intestinal obstruction [2, 3].

5.1. Distension

The distension of obstructed bowel above the obstacle is due to the accumulation of fluid and gas. The intestinal gas that normally progresses by peristaltic movements shows the following composition at the start of occlusion: swallowed air, carbon dioxide (it comes from neutralization of bicarbonates), and later on gas bacterial fermentation. The carbon dioxide that forms in large quantities in the intestinal cavity participates minimally gaseous accumulation because it is largely absorbed by the intestinal mucosa.

Nitrogen N_2	70%
Oxygen O_2	10–12%
Carbone dioxide CO_2	6–9%
Hydrogen H_2	1%
Methane CH_4	1%
Hydrogen disulphide	1–10%

Table 3. Intestinal obstruction: composition of intestinal gas.

On the contrary, the swallowed air significantly contributes to gaseous bowel distension because it contains a high rate of nitrogen content, which is not absorbed: in fact about 70% of the intestinal gas is constituted by nitrogen.

For this reason, the nasogastric aspiration in the patients with intestinal distension should be relevant and useful.

A little advantage can be added to gastric aspiration by the administration of pure oxygen to distended patients because increasing the pressure of a gas increases its solubility [4].

The common composition of intestinal gas in obstruction is reported in **Table 3** [5, 6].

5.2. Fluid loss

In the distended bowel above, the obstruction gastrointestinal secretions accumulate in large amounts. This occurs for two reasons: deprivation of the absorptive activity of intestine beyond the obstruction and also damage in fluid and electrolyte exchange in the wall of the obstructed and distended gut [7].

Source	Volume (ml)
Saliva	1500
Gastric secretion	2500
Bile	500
Pancreatic juice	700
Intestinal mucosa secretion	3000
Total	8200
Normal plasmatic volume	3500

Table 4. Volume of digestive secretion per day.

The saliva, gastric secretion, bile, pancreatic juice, and small intestinal secretion accumulate the total volume of about 8000 ml in 24 h as reported in more detail in **Table 4**. These fluid secretions are isotonique with the plasma, except for gastric secretion, which has minor sodium concentration (**Figure 3**) [8].

Therefore, normally water and electrolytes absorption is almost complete in the colon. In small bowel obstruction, the function of the colon cannot develop and the total intestinal secretions accumulate in the obstructed gut.

Beside the decreased absorption in the obstructed patients, there is also, above the obstacle, increased secretion into the bowel lumen.

In the pathophysiology of intestinal obstruction, the fluid and electrolytes loss plays a very important role. The progressive accumulation of gas and fluid in the intestinal lumen allows the increase in the endoluminal pressure to very high values: in the small bowel the pressure can reach 15 cm H_2O, whereas in the colon it can reach 25 cm H_2O. In the initial period of mechanical obstruction in the intestinal segments above the obstacle, active peristalsis causes further pressure rise to 20–30 cm H_2O [9]. In the large bowel, the intraluminal pressure can reach 50 cm H_2O because the pressure increase is based on the product of the pressure value multiplied by bowel diameter. The major detrimental effect of the progressive gut distension and intraluminal pressure increase is the impairment of the intramural circulation of the bowel.

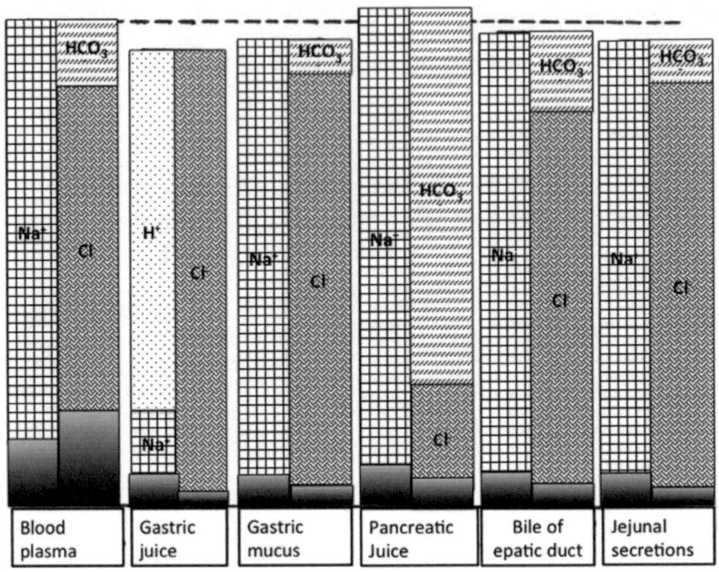

Figure 3. Electrolytes composition in blood plasma and digestive secretion.

5.3. Pathophysiology of circulatory changes in the distended bowel

The experimental studies demonstrated the linear connection between bowel obstruction, increase in intraluminal pressure, gut wall distension, changes in blood flow [10]. In the clinical situations, there are some difficulties to connect the degree of intraluminal pressure, intestinal distension, and the damage of parietal blood perfusion.

In the pathological setting, the increase in the intraluminal pressure should develop slowly and should not reach high degree [11, 12].

The intestinal wall distension in the obstructed patients causes increased distensibility of the gut wall that becomes more vulnerable to a further increment of distension. In this way, a small rise in the intraluminal pressure and the wall distension allows considerable tension in the intestinal wall and increased resistance in the capillaries with damage bowel blood flow.

The ischemic necrosis of obstructed bowel should be caused by progressive thinning of gut wall, reduction of the lumen of vessels, and finally interruption of the blood supply [4].

In the pathogenetic sequence, start a self-handing mechanism because the parietal distension increases the intestinal secretions with further intraluminal fluid accumulation, increased wall distension, impaired parietal blood flow, and finally hypovolemia.

The intestinal secretions enhance because the capillary leak increases the fluid flux to intestinal lumen [12, 13].

Beside fluid and electrolytes accumulation in the obstructed bowel, there is further fluid loss with vomiting. The metabolic effects of electrolytes and fluid loss, subtracted from the circulating blood volume and interstitial spaces, depend on the duration and site of obstruction. Proximal small bowel obstructions cause early and abundant vomiting with fluid, Cl, Na, and K loss, and consequently dehydration, hypokalemia, hyponatremia, hypochloremia, and metabolic alkalosis. In these proximal obstructions, the gut distension is less evident. On the contrary, the distal small bowel obstructions show more evident gut distension but the fluid and electrolytes depletion develop slowly, based on late vomiting and longer preserved resorption capacity. The dehydration causes hypovolemia, tachycardia, renal failure, decrease in the central venous pressure (CVP), and cardiac output, finally the hypovolemic shock. Moreover, the bowel distension may cause increase in the endoabdominal pressure with damage of venous return and pulmonary ventilation.

5.4. Bacteriology

Normally, the small intestine contains only transient bacterial flora with scanty growth because of the fluid content and fast transit. In fact, bacteria traverse the small intestine so rapidly that significant growth does not occur.

Instead in the case of obstruction and stasis, proliferation by geometrical progression results in rapid colonization of the intestinal lumen [14, 15].

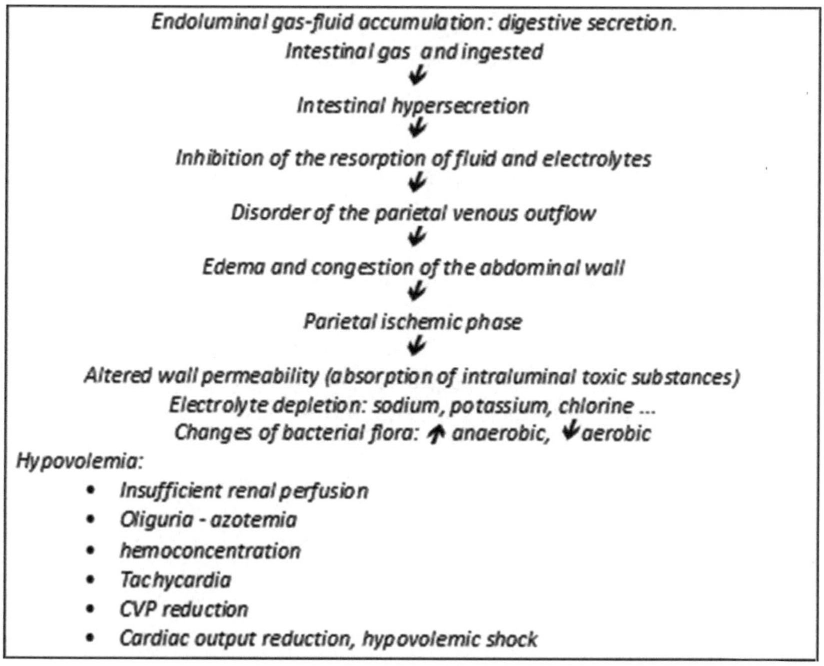

Figure 4. Intestinal obstruction: pathophysiological features.

Moreover, the increase in bacterial flora is particularly evident in the anaerobic organisms such as Bacteroides, Coliforms, and Clostridia [16]. The considerable increase in bacteria proliferation does not show clinical effects in the first phase of simple intestinal obstruction before the anatomical and functional impairment of intestinal wall.

The pathophysiological features in intestinal obstruction are summarized in **Figure 4**.

6. Pathophysiology of strangulation obstruction

The interruption of blood flow in an intestinal segment beside the lumen obstruction characterizes the strangulation obstruction. The most frequent causes of strangulation obstruction are incarcerated external hernias (abdominal wall: inguinal, femoral, umbilical, and incisional hernias), internal hernias (fibrous band, paraduodenal, foramen of Winslow, pericecal, intersigmoid, transmesenteric, and retroanastomotic), volvolus, and intussusception.

The pressure in the obstructed intestinal segment exceeds very quickly the pressure venous in the bowel wall and in the corresponding mesentery. The following step is the venous blockage in these vessels, then capillary rupture with hemorrhagic infarction in the submucosa, mucosa, and finally in all layers of intestinal wall.

The ischemic evolution of this condition is preceded by intramural thrombosis veins and is completed with the necrosis that proceeds from the mucosa to the serosa.

In the necrotic intestinal segment, the perforation can occur followed by severe septic peritonitis. Before this final lethal conclusion, the severe septic-toxic conditions can develop in the strangulation occlusion.

The damage of the blood supply and the normal function of intestinal wall allow serious consequences with transudation of toxic materials from Gram-positive and especially Gram-negative anaerobic organisms of intestinal obstructed lumen across the bowel wall in the peritoneal cavity. The systemic effects of the absorption by peritoneal serosa of toxic material are serious hemodynamic alterations, hypovolemia, hypotension, and septic shock. The role of intestinal bacterial flora in the production of the toxic transudation has been demonstrated in the past by Cohn, based on the protective action of antibiotics [17]. Beside the toxic systemic compromissions, in the strangulation obstruction, the metabolic consequences of fluid and electrolytes loss also develop such as in the simple intestinal obstruction.

7. Pathophysiology of large bowel obstruction

The pathophysiological syndrome of large bowel obstruction in general terms can be overlapped by small bowel obstruction but differs in the time in which it develops. The obstruction of the right colon is quite similar to distal small bowel obstruction in the pathophysiological evolution.

The distal large bowel obstructions (left, sigmoid colon, and rectum) instead show characteristic pathophysiological and clinical data.

Large bowel obstruction follows a slower course. The symptoms of dehydration are less severe. In the early stages, the colon retains the absorption capacity of fluid and electrolytes. For this reason, it preserves normal blood electrolyte concentration; therefore, the isotonic loss of water and electrolytes is associated with decreased plasma volume: hemoconcentration, decrease of CVP, and oliguria.

In the obstructed colon, the gaseous distension and the endoluminal pressure increase progressively. Consequently, it can develop damage of the blood flow in the parietal vessel earlier and more evident than in the small gut because the colon has the lowest blood flow across the abdominal viscera. The ischemia interests before the mucosa, impairing its functions; furthermore, this condition points out that the intraoperative evaluation of colonic blood perfusion cannot be based only on an external examination of serous membrane.

The increasing endoluminal pressure in the intestinal segment with thin walls, such as cecum, can cause perforation and septic peritonitis. Also in large bowel obstruction, the blockage of intestinal content increases the growth of bacterial flora, and the damage of intestinal wall functions allows the absorption of septic-toxic fluid intestinal content. In the beginning, only the colon is distended but usually the ileocecal valve becomes incompetent and allows the dilatation to progress proximally into the small gut. The presentation of the clinical picture of "closed-loop obstruction" without distension of small bowel that preserves its functions for a short period is quite unusual. This condition is due to competent ileocecal valve with a double obstruction, the valve and colonic obstruction, and the risk in the closed loop with an increase in the intraluminal pressure, obstruction of blood supply, gangrene, perforation, and peritonitis.

The obstructions of large bowel in the majority of cases are due to neoplastic diseases, adhesions, and volvulus.

In the large bowel obstruction, the cramping pain occurs longer than small bowel occlusion.

Colonic volvulus (cecal or sigmoid) are characterized by a great dilatation of cecum or sigmoid colon on imaging exams (plain radiography—CT scan). The neoplastic obstruction of distal colon or rectum shows great distension of the colon above the obstacle and chronic and progressive symptoms of constipation with the change of regular bowel function toward constipated bowel function, changes of stool caliber, long-term cathartic use. Abdominal CT scan can demonstrate a mass as a cause of large bowel obstruction and synchronous lesions as metastases and enlarged lymph nodes.

8. Pathophysiology of paralytic obstruction of the intestines (adynamic ileus)

There are distension and vomiting in this form of obstruction of the bowel but no mechanical obstruction. The adynamic ileus is due to a paralysis of the musculature of the bowel. Hypokalemia causes intracellular reduction of potassium that is replaced by sodium and consequently depolarization of electric potentials of membranes of muscle and nerve cells, which aggravates the intestinal paralysis.

Intestinal motility has dual adjustment, central and peripheral or autonomous: this explains the variability of causes and stimuli that provoke a reflex paresis of the intestinal musculature.

In fact, we have to consider peritonitis, retroperitoneal hemorrhage, renal trauma, renoureteral colic, lesions of dorsal-lumbar spine, pneumonia, and pleurisy basal, some neurological drugs, and finally the laparotomy causing a transient disturbance of gastrointestinal motility (postoperative dynamic ileus).

Distension is associated with altered motility to stabilize the occlusive syndrome. In the beginning, the distension stimulates the peristalsis, but, settled the occlusive conditions, with greater distension the inhibitory effect is largest. In fact, the gut distension causes the inhibitory reflex of intestinal motility by receptors of longitudinal musculature of the bowel.

The accumulation of fluid and gas is accompanied by altered functions of intestinal mucosa. Clinical presentation of adynamic ileus is usually less severe than mechanical obstruction.

Clinical findings are abdominal distension, the absence of flatus and bowel movement, and vomiting. There are no colicky pain and peristalsis because of the intestinal paralysis [18].

The basic radiologic examination shows intestinal distension and some air-fluid levels, i.e., messy. The radiological finding that can confirm the diagnosis of ileus is the air in the colon and rectum, and on abdominal computed tomography (CT), there is no demonstrable mechanical obstruction [19]. Usually, the therapeutic approach is conservative based on the control and improvement of fluid and electrolytes disorders, particularly hypokalemia. It can also be useful in some patients in controlling particular medication as opiates or anticholinergics.

9. Diagnosis

Different clinical forms are included in the generic diagnosis of "intestinal obstruction", which are to be distinguished from each other. Therefore, we propose a diagnostic course divided into sequential steps.

First, a preliminary diagnosis with distinction between simple versus strangulation obstruction is performed.

Then, in the first step of the diagnosis, the distinction of mechanical or paralytic obstruction is performed.

In the second step of diagnosis, we assess the level of obstruction, such as high small bowel obstruction, low small bowel obstruction, and large bowel obstruction.

Finally, in the third step of diagnosis, the type of obstacle is defined based on imaging examinations.

Each data (history, physical examination, laboratory, and instrumental) of the diagnostic evaluation could take on particular characteristic useful for a precise differential diagnosis, such as simple obstruction, strangulation, large bowel obstruction, and so on.

In the history, some data are relevant to the risk of bowel obstruction. Prior abdominal or pelvic surgery and peritoneal sepsis can cause adhesions and bands following any operations or septic process in the abdomen.

The evaluation should be made of inflammatory bowel disease (IBD) or other intestinal inflammation based on the previous diagnosis, therapy, and evolution of the disease.

History and current evolution of gastrointestinal or gynecologic neoplasms previously treated with surgery, chemotherapy, and irradiation can be risk factors for intestinal obstruction.

Most relevant in the history should be the communication of the change in regularity and frequency of bowel movement by an elderly patient due to possibility of undiagnosed colorectal cancer. Clinical features of intestinal obstruction are especially focused on two symptoms and two signs: colicky abdominal pain, absence of flatus or bowel movements, abdominal distension, and vomiting.

Abdominal pain is colicky, cramping, due to increased peristalsis, with paroxysms occurring every 4–5 min. In the first phase of obstruction, the abdominal pain should be more severe but if it is prolonged the occlusion for a serious delay in therapy can reduce the intensity of pain because peristalsis stops, so its disappearance should be a bad sign. In the later phase, it also increases abdominal distension and fluid—electrolytes loss [20, 21].

Periumbilical and cramping pain can be due to distal small bowel obstruction. Proximal small bowel obstruction could develop with less pain and distension but severe vomiting.

Large bowel obstruction (especially distal colon) may show pain below umbilicus and the paroxysms may occur longer for intervals of 6–10 min.

Severe and continuous pain should suggest strangulation obstruction. The absence of flatus and bowel movement in the true intestinal obstruction is complete. If there is small bowel obstruction, colon may take 1 or 2 days to empty. Indeed, the obstructive syndrome starts with the absence of flatus. The vomiting in the high, proximal small bowel obstruction is profuse and frequent. The higher is the obstruction, the worse is the vomiting. In the large bowel or distal small bowel obstruction, the vomiting can be delayed. After about 3 days of complete obstruction, the vomiting becomes feculent because the change in the intestinal bacterial flora causes a significant increase in anaerobic organisms. In the large bowel, obstruction may appear early vomiting reflex type based on intestinal distension. Abdominal distension should be considered the most frequent physical sign of intestinal obstruction [22–24].

The degree of abdominal distension varies depending upon the site of the obstacle or the extension of the obstructed bowel. In the proximal, small gut occlusion could occur at a lower degree of abdominal distension or no distension: intestinal occlusion without distension. In distal small bowel or large bowel obstruction, the abdominal distension is the most obvious clinical relevance. Abdominal distension is also present and obvious in the patients with dynamic obstruction or intestinal pseudo-obstruction. If distension is conspicuous and other signs are minimal, there is probably large gut obstruction. Sigmoid volvulus can cause extreme distension. On the other hand, in the first phase of obstructive syndrome, the patients with a "closed-loop obstruction" or intestinal hernias or small bowel volvulus with short intestinal segment, abdominal distension can be minimal.

Beside the abdominal distension, the physical examination can point out hyperresonance, obstructive gut sounds, and visible peristalsis.

In the obstructed patients, it is possible to hear some characteristic sounds by abdominal auscultation: runs of borborygmi, chorus of tinkling high pitched musical sounds at the same time of peristaltic waves, and colicky pain. These data by auscultation are absent in the patients with abdominal distension by dynamic occlusion. Distended bowel results in hyperresonance or tympany to abdominal percussion, but fluid-filled loops can result in dullness. The visible peristalsis can be seen in very thin patients.

Simple obstruction	Strangulation obstruction
	Evidence of abdominal wall incarcerated hernias (groin, femoral, and obturator incisional)
Colicky pain Absent abdominal tenderness	Fast onset of abdominal pain. Constant pain, not colicky. Abdominal tenderness localized or diffuse
	Finally, peritoneal signs due to peritonitis (bowel ischemia, perforation, and peritonitis)

Table 5. Intestinal obstruction: preliminary differential diagnosis.

	Mechanical	Dynamic
History	Previous abdominal or pelvic surgery, radiation therapy, history of abdominal malignancy	Every risk factors of dynamic occlusion (causes of reflex paresis)
Pain	Present, colicky	Absent or due to abdominal distension
Vomiting	Present	Present
Abdominal distension	Present	Present
Absence of flatus or bowel movement	Present	Present
Plain radiography	Bowel distention Evident air-fluid levels differential height, regular arranged disposition	Bowel distention. Few air-fluid levels—somewhat messy

Table 6. Intestinal obstruction: first steps differential diagnosis.

The clinical examination should evaluate systemic compromission of intestinal obstruction syndrome. It should be highlighted dehydration, tachycardia, hypotension, reduced urine output, fever, electrolytes alterations, and dry mucus membranes. The physical examination of abdomen will be completed with control of old laparotomy scar, any abdominal wall, or groin hernias.

The examination can identify the abnormal masses, such as abscess, volvulus, and tumor, which can be the cause of obstruction. Abdominal tenderness is not a characteristic feature of uncomplicated obstruction. Obvious tenderness localized or diffuse suggests complicated obstruction: strangulation, perforation, etc.

Rectal examination is an integral part of a clinical examination. Usually, this examination cannot add further information but it can find rectal neoplastic lesion or mucus or blood that probably suggests a strangulating lesion higher up, intussusception, or inflammatory intestinal lesion such as IBD.

Based on the clinical appearance and basic radiological examinations, the first steps of the diagnosis are shown in **Tables 5–7**.

	High small bowel occlusion	Low small bowel occlusion	Large bowel occlusion
Pain	Absent	Evident	Evident
Vomiting	Early, copious, continuous	Late	Very late
Abdominal distension	Absent	Present	Present
Absence of flatus or bowel movement	Present	Present	Present
Plain radiography	Is it possible follow the distended bowel segments and hypotize the site of obstruction (transition between dilated proximal and non-dilated distal bowel)		

Table 7. Intestinal obstruction: second-step differential diagnosis.

9.1. Laboratory studies

Routine laboratory studies are not specific for a diagnosis of intestinal obstruction. The laboratory data should evaluate hypovolemia, initial renal failure, hemoconcentration, metabolic abnormalities (hyponatremia, hypokalemia), and leucocytosis.

Neutrophylic leucocytosis can signalize complications such as strangulation or ischemic lesions. On the other hand, the anemia can indicate intestinal tumor or IBD.

In the obstructed patients with appearance of systemic compromission (hypothermia, tachycardia, fever, and renal failure), the complete clinical assessment requires arterial blood gas (ABG) and serum lactate. These evaluations can show some different details. Metabolic alkalosis follows severe vomiting. Metabolic acidosis takes place in the case of severe hypovolemia, hypoperfusion, organ failure, and ischemic bowel lesions [25]. The laboratory markers of ischemia to differentiate simple bowel obstruction from strangulation obstruction have been long searched [26]. First, elevated serum lactate (metabolic acidosis) with not very high specificity (sensitivity 90%, specificity 87%) can be used [27, 28]. Cronk et al. has suggested the use, as marker of ischemia with valuable results, of intestinal fatty acid binding protein, connected to necrotic enterocytes [29].

The third step of our assessment of intestinal obstruction can allow the achievement of more defined diagnosis.

9.2. Plain radiography

About some imaging modalities, plain radiography is mostly employed. This is very practical and useful because it can confirm basic diagnosis of intestinal obstruction [30]. Usually, there are only few data useful for the distinction between mechanical or dynamic obstruction. Moreover, the plain radiography is widely available and less expensive; its regular performance requires an upright position of patients; the lateral position is a makeshift solution. The supine position shows insufficient results for diagnosis, only bowel distension. The findings of plain radiography in bowel obstruction are as follows:

- Multiple air fluid levels, more evident based on upright position;
- Dilatation of intestinal segments proximal the obstacle and collapse in distal bowel.

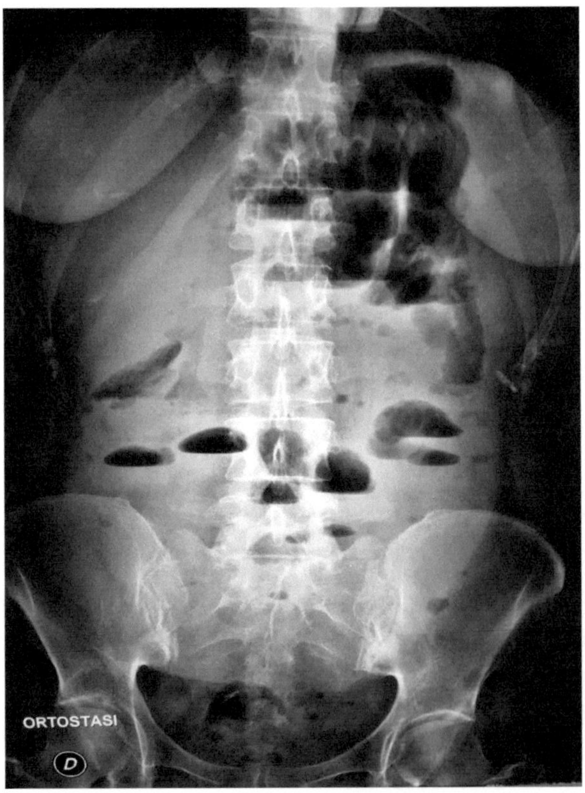

Figure 5. Plain radiography: small bowel obstruction.

These can be useful for the diagnosis of mechanical obstruction: the remark of a regular arranged disposition of multiple air fluid levels with evident size increases from each other (**Figure 5**) [31]. The plain radiography can detect the pneumoperitoneum by intestinal perforation. We have to remember that the remark of less gaseous distension (gasless abdomen) of intestinal loops in obstructed patients can be possible because of a complete fluid filling of loops. Mullaw suggests the evaluation of the string of pearls sign: fluid-filled bowel loops with small amounts of intraluminal gas [32]. Certainly, plain abdominal radiography in upright position can confirm the basic diagnosis of intestinal obstruction with high enough sensitivity (80%) and specificity (75%) [33]. The use of the examination in detecting the site of obstacle and in differentiating the small from large bowel obstruction is very limited.

9.3. Abdominal CT

Plain abdominal films, normally upright position if possible, should be the first imaging examination in the diagnostic program of suspected intestinal obstruction because it is readily available and in some cases it is resolvable if the doubt of obstruction is not confirmed. However, normally we must complete the diagnosis with abdominal CT scan. The performance of CT in the diagnostic plan is now valuable. Some data are similar to the findings of plain radiography as bowel dilatation above the obstruction and air-fluid levels. CT scan usually can identify the specific site of obstruction clarifying the transition point of distended and empty loops and also the complete intestinal occlusion. This examination should detect the etiology of obstruction by identifying internal or parietal hernias, neoplastic or inflammatory masses, and recognize the complications such as ischemic/necrotic evolution over all by strangulation obstruction and finally the perforation [32, 34–36]. CT scan can provide other diagnostic information: ascites, rotation of mesentery (whirl sign), mesenteric edema, bowel wall thickening >3 mm, submucosal edema-hemorrhage, venous cutoff sign by venous thrombosis, poor segmental bowel wall enhancement, pneumomatosis intestinalis, edematous mesentery, and hemorrhage in the mesentery. All these findings can suggest complications that have vascular involvement in intestinal obstruction [37–39].

9.4. Abdominal ultrasonography

Abdominal US is now considered as an integral part of clinical examination and consequently it is currently performed in the patients with abdominal pains. Finally, it can be employed in the patients with contraindications to CT, pregnant patients, and patients with very severe systemic impairment. The contribution of abdominal US to intestinal obstruction diagnosis should be limited to identify intestinal distension, abdominal masses, and internal hernias, which can be site of incarcerated intestinal loops. Abdominal US can provide very few findings about air-fluid levels, the site, etiology, and complications of intestinal obstruction [40].

9.5. MRI

The accuracy of magnetic resonance imaging (MRI) is almost similar to CT scan for the confirmation of basic diagnosis of obstructions, location, and etiology of the obstruction. This examination shows poor detection of masses and inflammation [41–43].

Contrast studies, such as water soluble contrast material or contrast fluoroscopy, have indications and purposes rather limited in the obstruction diagnosed as complete and persistent.

10. Management

The first approach in the management of intestinal obstruction includes the correction of physiologic impairment caused by obstruction. Some measures can be required: the use of a bladder catheter to monitoring urine output, adequate intravenous access, arterial canalization, and CVP monitoring.

The purpose of the therapeutic approach is the correction of hypovolemia and electrolytes depletion with volume resuscitation. The development of fluid-electrolyte replacement and the adequacy of resuscitation should be guided by the degree of systemic impairment and the reaction of the patient to therapy. Therefore, aggressive replacement of fluid and electrolytes can be employed after restoration of renal function. The use of nasogastric tube for the control of severe intestinal distension can be helpful.

Antibiotics should be started at the confirmation of diagnosis of intestinal obstruction, mostly if fever, and leucocytosis is present.

The aim of the use of antibiotics is based on the control and treatment of intestinal overgrowth of bacteria and their translocation across the bowel wall [44].

Antibiotics, based on the particular type of bacterial overgrowth in the obstruction, could have more coverage against anaerobes and Gram-negative bacteria. The main objective of the therapeutic program of bowel obstruction is to remove the obstacle. Surgery is the leading option.

Three criteria guide this therapeutic choice:

- Degree of impairment of general conditions due to complications: intestinal ischemia, necrosis, perforation, and peritonitis;
- Etiology of obstructive syndrome (hypothesized or confirmed);
- Type of intestinal obstruction diagnosed (hypothesized or confirmed):
- Complete versus incomplete
- Small or large bowel obstacle site
- Strangulation occlusion

Peritonitis and abdominal sepsis caused by complications of obstructive syndrome (perforation, ischemia, necrosis, etc.) prescribe urgent surgical intervention. The choices of the surgical procedures are conditioned by pathological findings, sometimes intraoperative.

Clinical instability, diagnostic uncertainly, unexplained leucocytosis and metabolic acidosis, and consequently the doubt of perforation or abdominal sepsis justify the abdominal surgical

http://dx.doi.org/10.5772/63156

exploration. Also the suspicion of strangulation occlusion, based on continuous and severe abdominal pains, should prompt surgery.

The surgical choice for irreducible or strangulated hernia of abdominal wall is very obvious.

In the case of high suspicion for digestive malignancy, most frequently in large bowel, surgical intervention should be performed. In these cases, surgical procedures should contemporary treat both diseases, intestinal obstruction and digestive neoplasm: primary resection followed by temporary diversion (Hartmann procedure) or immediate reconstruction.

In summary, for the complete and permanent intestinal obstruction, the surgical intervention should be the first-line option.

In the management of intestinal obstructions, there are some issues under discussion with no simple solution.

The treatment of acute small bowel obstruction should be a common clinical challenge. The choice of operative management within the first 12–24 h from the onset can be followed by nontherapeutic laparotomy with the unfortunate results of further adhesions and postoperative morbidities [45]. Nasogastric decompression, fluid-electrolytes replacement, and careful clinical reassessment can have a considerable success rate in the approach of small bowel obstruction. Unfortunately, failure to acknowledge or late recognition of strangulation obstruction cause increased morbidity and mortality [46–48]. In this complicated setting, the solution is the selection of the patients. Of course, as stated previously, the cases with clinical and/or instrumental evidence of peritoneal phlogosis or perforation are excluded from this evaluation. Some criteria have been proposed to identify the patients with alleged simple small bowel obstruction for immediate operative treatment. Clinical appearance of fast onset of abdominal pain, continuous pain, not colicky, abdominal tenderness localized, or diffuse on physical examination suggest the choice of immediate surgical approach. There are also specific findings on abdominal CT: free intraperitoneal fluid, mesenteric edema, thickened wall, pneumatosis intestinalis, "small bowel feces signs" (gas bubbles and debris within the lumen of obstructed small bowel) [49]. On the other hand, the selected patients' choice for nonoperative management should be characterized by the following criteria: the absence of abdominal wall hernias, previous abdominal pelvic surgery, previous abdominal malignancies, history and diagnosis of IBD (especially Crohn disease), colicky pain, absent abdominal tenderness on clinical assessment, and finally hemodynamic stability and absence of impairment of general conditions.

In summary, clinically stable patients with partial obstruction can be treated by conservative management [50].

Conservative management includes intestinal intubation and decompression, aggressive intravenous rehydration, and antibiotics [51].

The results of the conservative management of acute mechanical small bowel obstruction are uncertain and not conclusive, from the data of literature [52]. There are high success rates in the stable patients with incomplete obstruction [53, 54]. Among the patients with adhesive small bowel obstruction, 24.6% of patients are treated with nonoperative management, without surgery or readmission [55]. On the other hand, high rates of recurrence and the risk of complications including vascular impairment were reported [47]. Therefore, among the patients managed conservatively to start with, the operative rates were very high because of the diagnostic difficulty to distinguish simple from strangulation obstruction on clinical and instrumental examinations [56].

The international guidelines [34, 57] for the evaluation and management of small bowel obstruction confirm and summarize the data from the literature.

The guidelines in evidence are as follows:

- The instrumental diagnosis should be based on the CT scan of abdomen because it can clarify the grade, severity, and etiology of small bowel obstruction.
- Urgent surgical approach is the first option for small bowel obstructions with evidence of peritonitis or clinical deterioration (fever, tachycardia, leucocytosis, and metabolic acidosis).
- Patients with partial or complete small bowel obstruction and stable general conditions and without physical and instrumental signs of peritoneal phlogosis can undergo initial nonoperative management.
- Water-soluble contrast study can be useful in partial small bowel obstruction not resolved within 48 h based on the improvement of water-soluble contrast on bowel function.
- After 3–5 days of conservative management, the patients with small bowel obstruction should undergo surgery;
- Laparoscopic treatment can be a safe and possible procedure for small bowel obstruction, but not commonly employed. In fact, its use requires some selection criteria: proximal obstruction, localized distension on radiography, no sepsis, and mild abdominal distension [58–60].

Large bowel obstruction due to colorectal cancer requires the treatment of malignancy and abdominal urgency. The first objective should be the control and management of malignancy. Several factors may influence the therapeutic choice: the location of the tumor (proximal-distal colon), the degree of colonic distension and the impairment of blood flow of intestinal wall, the involvement of the general conditions of the patient with organ failure, dehydration, hypovolemia, and sepsis.

In this scenario, variable and complex, it is very difficult to establish a well-defined and unequivocal line therapy in relation to the surgical procedure to be used. There are several proposals: at the beginning resolution of the occlusive complication only with colostomy (two-stage procedure) followed, sometime later, by resection of neoplastic lesion (with radical surgical criteria or palliative). On the other hand, a one-stage procedure with resection of the tumor (radical or palliative), followed by temporary colostomy (Hartmann's procedure) or primary anastomosis, can be employed.

Endoscopic colonic stents have been proposed in neoplastic obstruction of distal colon for palliation or as a bridge to surgery [61]. With the palliative intent, the colorectal stent can be used as an alternative to colostomy, whereas in the hospitals it can be employed as a bridge to elective surgery with specific expertise [62].

The tumor site along the colon is an important factor for the therapeutic choice. Right colectomy can be defined as the treatment of choice for right-sided colon cancer in obstruction setting. It is a safe technique for one-stage resection and anastomosis [63]. The guidelines of World Society of Emergency Surgery suggest some recommendations on obstructive left colon carcinoma [62]. Hartmann's procedure should be the preferred choice in the patients with impaired blood supply of intestinal wall and high surgical risk compared to loop colostomy. Hartmann's procedure shows overlapped survival results compared to segmental colonic resection with primary anastomosis.

The patients submitted to primary resection and anastomosis have similar mortality-morbidity rates with total or subtotal colectomy and segmental colectomy. The immediate results are similar in these patients (with primary resection and anastomosis) related to the choice of intraoperative colonic irrigation or manual decompression.

11. Intestinal pseudo-obstruction

Intestinal pseudo-obstruction is a syndrome characterized by a complete intestinal dilatation, generally of large bowel, without mechanical obstacle. The proposal nosography of intestinal pseudo-obstruction is reported in **Table 8**.

Intestinal pseudo-obstruction
Acute
Hydro electrolytes alterations
Anticholinergic, ganglionic blocker drugs
Laparotomy
Intraperitoneal diseases (perforation, appendicitis, cholecystitis, pancreatitis)
Extraperitoneal diseases (hematoma, vertebral trauma, pneumonia, myocardial infarct)
Sclerosing therapy of esophagus
Acute colonic pseudo-obstruction
Chronic
Secondary
Endocrine disease (diabetes, hypothyroidism)
Collagenopathies (scleroderma, dermatomyositis)
Neuropathies (Parkinson's disease, multiple sclerosis)
Degenerative diseases (amyloidosis)
Elevated blood levels of prostaglandin A, E, F
Idiopathic
Hereditary hollow visceral myopathy
Familiar neuronal disease

Table 8. Intestinal pseudo-obstruction: nosography.

The intestinal pseudo-obstruction can affect small or large bowel and it may be possible to differentiate the syndromes with acute or chronic onset and evolution.

Paralytic ileus can be inserted in the broader field of acute pseudo-obstructions that are based on pathophysiological impairment of intestinal peristalsis (intestinal paresis). The acute pseudo-obstruction can be caused by severe fluid electrolytes disorders (hypokalemia, hypocalcemia), medications with anticholinergics or opiates, abdominal interventions (postoperative ileus), inflammatory and septic abdominal diseases as peritonitis, pancreatitis, perforations, intestinal ischemia, and retroperitoneal trauma.

In this area, the acute colonic pseudo-obstruction (ACPO) (Ogilvie's syndrome) should be highlighted. The Ogilvie's syndrome has been diagnosed in association with various pathologies such as cholecystitis, acute pancreatitis, retroperitoneal traumatic hematoma, Parkinson disease, and so on. The impaired colonic motility should be caused by imbalance in the autonomic nervous system: increase in sympathetic tone and decrease in parasympathetic tone [64]. Increased sympathetic tone to the colon results in the inhibition of colonic motility [65]. The pathologic findings, more evident in the right colon, are distension, fluid-gaseous accumulation, and increased endoluminal pressure. Severe blood circulatory impairment can occur in the large bowel wall with damage of venous return, edema, trophic mucosal alteration to serous, sometimes necrosis, and perforation. The cecum is more dilated colonic section. According to Laplace's law, the cecum, with its larger diameter, requires less pressure to increase in size and in wall tension. Ischemia, longitudinal splitting of serosa, and herniation of the mucosa and perforation, the so-called "diastasis breaking" of cecum, is caused with the increased wall tension.

Clinical features are obvious abdominal distension as earliest sign, no tenderness, hyperresonance, or tympany to percussion throughout the abdomen, and no peristalsis and bowel sounds to auscultation. The symptoms are similar to large bowel obstruction and develop over 3–7 days.

Imaging examinations, plain radiography, CT scan should help to exclude mechanical bowel obstruction. The size of the cecum (more than 8–10 mm) on abdominal films could be useful to decide colonic decompression, surgical or endoscopic, because of the risk of perforation [66].

In the ACPO, conservative treatment can be proposed: no oral intake, nasogastric decompression, correction of fluid and electrolytes disorders, and discontinuance of drugs that inhibit gastrointestinal motility [67].

In the conservative option, the use of pharmacologic agents can be added to increase colonic motility. Several drugs have been employed with nonunique and uncertain results, erytromicin, cisapride, metoclopramide, and neostigmine [68, 69]. The invasive therapeutic approach of Ogilvie's syndrome includes colonoscopic decompression and surgical intervention. The endoscopic decompression should be a safe and effective procedure for ACPO and has been associated with high success rates (77–86%) [70].

Recurrence rates of colonoscopy decompression are also high, ranging from 20 to 60% [71]. Clinical signs of ischemia, abdominal sepsis, perforation, or failure of conservative management require surgery. The choice of surgical procedure is indicated by intraoperative pathological findings: tube cecostomy, subtotal colectomy, etc.

Chronic intestinal pseudo-obstruction can be subdivided into secondary and idiopathic. In the first cases, the chronic pseudo-obstructions are part of severe systemic diseases: endocrine diseases (diabetes and hypothyroidism) and collagenopathies (scleroderma, amyloidosis, dermatomyositis, and lupus erythematosus). The chronic intestinal idiopathic pseudo-obstructions are frequently familiar diseases. Pathophysiology is not completely defined and should be based on derangement of autonomic nervous system with alteration of intestinal motility. The pathophysiological findings are hereditary hollow visceral myopathy, familiar neuronal visceral disease, lesion of myenteric plexus, and alimentary tract ganglioneuromatosis.

The role of interstitial cells of Cajal has been hypothesized in the pathogenesis of idiopathic chronic intestinal pseudo-obstruction. Electron microscopy and immunochemistry studies showed a decreased number of interstitial cells of Cajal in the intestinal wall and alterations in interstitial cells of Cajal network [72].

According to clinical features, the cramping abdominal pain is more frequent; nausea, vomiting, and abdominal distension are occasional, sporadic. There are also alternating diarrhea and constipation and weight loss. Finally, the clinical evolution of the disease is chronic.

The results of the therapy of secondary forms are scantly and uncertain; usually, the therapy is connected with the treatment of the serious systemic diseases. Drugs that stimulate the smooth muscles (acetylcolinesterase inhibitors) can be employed in the idiopathic forms. Surgical procedures are indicated for the treatment of severe and continuous symptomatology that can be related to a portion of the digestive tract or for complete failure of conservative therapy [73].

Acknowledgements

The author is very grateful to Drs Libero Luca Giambavicchio and Francesco Lapolla for their valuable assistance in the typographical transcription of the manuscript.

Author details

Vincenzo Neri

Address all correspondence to: vincenzo.neri@unifg.it

General Surgery, University of Foggia, Foggia, Italy

References

[1] Miller G, Boman J, Shirier I et al. Etiology of small bowel obstruction. Am J Surg. 2000;180:33–36.

[2] Kozol R. Mechanical bowel obstruction: a tale of 2 eras. Arch Surg. 2012; 147:180.

[3] Wangensteen OH. Understanding the bowel obstruction problem. Am J Surg. 1978; 135: 131–149.

[4] Ellis H. Intestinal obstruction. Pathology. New York: Appleton – Century – Crofts.; 1982. p. 11–19.

[5] Duthie HL. Intestine. In: Irvine WT, editor. The scientific basis of surgery. 82nd ed. London: Churchill Livingstone; 1972.

[6] Grimble G. Fibre, fermentation, flora and flatus. GUT. 1989;20:6–13.

[7] Cappell MS, Batke M. Mechanical obstruction of the small bowel and colon. Med Clin North Am. 2008;92(3):575–597.

[8] Gamble JL. The companionship of water and electrolytes in the organization of body fluids. In: Lane medical lectures. Stanford: Stanford University Press; 1951.

[9] Camilleri M. Jejunal manometry in distal subacute mechanical obstruction: significance of prolonged simultaneous contractions. GUT 1989;30:468–475.

[10] Ohman V. Studies on small intestinal obstruction. Blood circulation in obstructed and artificially distended small intestine in the cat. Acta Chir Scand (Suppl). 1975;452:1–41.

[11] Wells C. Ileus and postoperative intestinal motility. Lancet. 1961;2:136–137.

[12] Wright HK, O'Brien JJ, Tilson MD. Water absorption in experimental closed segment obstruction of the ileum in man. Am J Surg. 1971;121;96–99.

[13] Shields R. The absorption and secretion of fluid and electrolytes by the obstructed bowel. Br J Surg. 1965;25:774.

[14] Bishop RF, Allock EA. Bacterial flora of the small intestine in acute intestinal obstruction Br Med J. 1960;1:766–770.

[15] Rana SV, Bhardwaj SB. Small intestinal bacteria overgrowth. Scand J Gastroenterol. 2008;43:1030–1037.

[16] Sykes PA, Bowlter KH, Schofield PF. The microflora of the obstructed bowel. Br J Surg. 1976;63:721–725.

[17] Cohn I. The "toxin" in "closed-loop" strangulation obstruction. Bull NY Acad Med. 1964;40:863–870.

[18] Batke M, Cappell MS. Adynamic ileus and acute colonic pseudo-obstruction. Med Clin North Am. 2008;92(3):649–670.

[19] Frager DH, Baer JW, Rothpearl H et al. Distinction between postoperative ileus and mechanical small bowel obstruction: value of CT compared with clinical and other radiographic findings. AJR Am J Roetgenol. 1995;164:891–894.

[20] Flasar MH, Goldberg E. The characteristics of abdominal pain could suggest some details of the diagnosis. Acute abdominal pain. Med Clin North Am. 2006;90:481.

[21] Irvin TT. Abdominal pain: a surgical audit of 1190 emergency admissions. Br J Surg. 1989:7b:1121–1125.

[22] Markogiannakis H, Messaris E, Dardamanis D et al. Acute mechanical bowel obstruction: clinical presentation, aetiology, management and outcome. World J Gastroenterol. 2007;13:432–437.

[23] Cheadle WG, Garr EE, Richardson JD. The importance of early diagnosis of small bowel obstruction. Am Surg. 1988;54:565–569.

[24] Perea Garcia J, Turegano Fuentes T, Quijada Garcia B et al. Adhesive small bowel obstruction: predictive value of oral contrast administration on the need for surgery. Rev Espan Enferm Dig. 2004;96:191–200.

[25] Takenkhi K, Tsuzuki Y, Ando T et al. Clinical studies of strangulating small bowel obstruction. Am Surg. 2004;70:40–44.

[26] Guzman-de la Garza FJ, Ibarra-Hernandez JM, Cordero-Perez P et al. Temporal relationship of serum markers and tissue damage during acute intestinal ischemia/reperfusion. Clinics (Sao Paulo). 2013;68:1034–1038.

[27] Murray MJ, Gonze MD, Nowak LR et al. Serum d(−)lactate levels as an aid to diagnosing acute intestinal ischemia. Am J Surg. 1994;167:575–578.

[28] Lange H, Jarkel R. Usefulness of plasma lactate concentration in the diagnosis of acute abdominal disease. Eur J Surg. 1994;160:381–384.

[29] Cronk DR, Houseworth TP, Cuadrado DG et al. Intestinal fatty acid binding protein (I-FABP) for the detection of strangulated mechanical small bowel obstruction. Curr Surg. 2006;63:322–325.

[30] Maglinte DD, Heitkamp DE, Howard TJ et al. Current concepts in imaging of small bowel obstruction. Radiol Clin North Am. 2003;41:263–283.

[31] Thompson WM, Kilani RK, Smit BB et al. Accuracy of abdominal radiography in acute small bowel obstruction: does reviewer experience matter? AJR Am J Roetgenol. 2007;188(33):233–238.

[32] Mullan CP, Siewert B, Eisenberg RL. Small bowel obstruction. AJR Am J Roetgenol. 2012;198(2):105–117.

[33] Suri S, Gupta S, Sudhakan PJ et al. Comparative evaluation of plain films, ultrasound and CT in the diagnosis of intestinal obstruction. Acta Radiol. 1999;40:422–428.

[34] Catena F, Di Saverio S, Kelly MD et al. Bologna guidelines for diagnosis and management of adhesive small bowel obstruction (ASBO): 2010 evidence-based Guidelines of the World Society of Emergency Surgery. World J Emerg Surg. 2011;6:5.

[35] Soyer P, Dohan A, Evenoc et al. Carcinoid tumors of the small bowel: evaluation with 64-section CT-enteroclysis. Eur J Radiol. 2015;82:943–950.

[36] Gong JS, Kang WY, Liu T et al. CT findings of a gastrointestinal stromal tumor arising from small bowel. Quant Imaging Med Surg. 2012;2:57–58.

[37] Ho YC. "Venous cut-off sign" as an adjunct to the "whirl sign" in recognizing acute small bowel volvulus via CT scan. J Gastroenterol Surg. 2012;16:2005–2006.

[38] Duda JB, Bhatt S, Dogra vs. utility of CT "whirl sign" in guiding management of small bowel obstruction. AJR AM J Roetgenol. 2008;191:743–747.

[39] Zalcman M, Sy M, Donckier V et al. Helical CT signs in the diagnosis of intestinal ischemia in small bowel obstruction. AJR Am J Roetgenol. 2000;175:1601–1607.

[40] Jang TB, Schindler D, Kaji AH. Bedside ultrasonography for the detection of small bowel obstruction in the emergency department. Emerg Med J. 2011;28:676–678.

[41] Diaz JJ Jr, Bokhari F, Mowery NT et al. Guidelines for management of small bowel obstruction. J Trauma. 2008;64:1651–1664.

[42] Kim JH, Ha HK, Sohn MJ et al. Usefulness of MR imaging for disease of small intestine: comparison with CT. Korean J Radiol. 2000;1:43–50.

[43] Beall DP, Fortman BJ, Lawler BC et al. Imaging bowel obstruction: a comparison between fast management resonance imaging and helical computed tomography. Clin Radiol. 2002;57:719–724.

[44] Sagar PM, MacFie J, Sedman P et al. Intestinal obstruction promotes gut translocation of bacteria. Dis Colon Rectum. 1995;38:640–644.

[45] Laws HL, Aldrete JS. Small bowel obstruction: a review of 465 cases. South Med J. 1976;69:733–734.

[46] Bickell NA, Federman AD, Aufses AH. Influence of time on risk of bowel resection in complete small bowel obstruction. J Am Coll Surg. 2005;201:847–854.

[47] Fevang BT, Jensen D, Svanes K et al. Early operation on conservative management of patients with small bowel obstruction? Eur J Surg. 2002;168:475–481.

[48] Shrock TR. Small intestine. In: Way LW, editor. Current surgical diagnosis and treatment. Norwalk, CT: Appleton and Large;1988. p. 561–585.

[49] Zielinski MD, Eiken PW, Bannon ME et al. Small bowel obstruction. Who needs an operation? A multivariate prediction model. World J Surg. 2010;34:910–919.

[50] Bauer J, Keeley B, Krieger B et al. Adhesive small bowel obstruction: early operative vs observational management. Am Surg. 2015;81:614–620.

[51] Chen SC, Yen ZS, Lee CC et al. Non surgical management of partial adhesive small bowel obstruction with oral therapy: a randomized controlled trial. CMAJ. 2005;173:1165–1169.

[52] Jackson PG, Raiji M. Evaluation and management of intestinal obstruction. Am Fam Phys. 2011;83:159–165.

[53] Mosley JG, Shoaib A. Operative versus conservative management of adhesional intestinal obstruction. Br J Surg. 2000;87:362–373.

[54] Williams SB, Greenspon J, Young HA et al. Small bowel obstruction: conservative vs surgical management. Dis Colon Rectum. 2005;48:1140–1146.

[55] Bauer J, Keelev B, Krieger B et al. Adhesive small bowel obstruction: early operative versus observational management. Am Surg. 2015;81:614–620.

[56] Khan TS, Wani SN et al. Clinico-pathological profile and management of acute mechanical small bowel obstruction: a prospective study. Arch Clin Exp Surg. 2013;2:154–160.

[57] Mang AA, Johnson DC, Piper GL et al. Evaluation and management of small bowel obstruction: an Eastern Association for surgery of trauma practice management guideline. J Trauma Acute Care Surg. 2012;73(5):5362–5369.

[58] Duk QY. Small bowel obstruction. Touli J, Gossot D, Hunter JG, editors. Endosurgery.New York: Churchill Livingstone; 1998. p. 425–431.

[59] Cirocchi R, Abraha I, Farinella E et al. Laparoscopic versus open surgery in small bowel obstruction. Cochrane Database Syst Rev. 2010;17(2);CD007511 [Review].

[60] Levard H, Boudet MJ, Msika S et al. Frenc Association for Surgical Research. Laparoscopic treatment of acute small bowel obstruction: a multicenter retrospective study. Anst NZ J Surg. 2001;71:641–646.

[61] Harris GJC, Senagore AJ, Lavary IC et al. The management of neoplastic colorectal obstruction with colonic endoluminal stenting devices. Am J Surg. 2001;181:499–506.

[62] Ansaloni L, Andersson RE, Bazzoli F et al. Guidelines in the management of obstructing cancer of the left colon: consensus conference of the World Society of Emergency Surgery (WSES) and Peritoneum and Surgery (PnS) Society. World J Emerg Surg. 2010;5:29.

[63] Frago R, Ramirez E, Millan M et al. Current management of acute malignant large bowel obstruction: a systematic review. Am J Surg. 2014;207:127–138.

[64] Manten HD, Pseudo-obstruction. Hanbrich WS, Schaffer F, Berk JF, editors. Bokus gastroenterology, vol. 2. Philadelphia: WB Saunders Co.; 1995. p. 1249–1267.

[65] Lee JT, Taylor BM, Singleton BC. Epidural anesthesia for acute pseudo-obstruction of the colon (Ogilvie's syndrome). Dis Colon Rectum. 1988;31:686–691.

[66] Edelman DA, Antaki F, Basson MD et al. Ogilvie Syndrome and Herpes zoster: case report and review of literature. J Emerg Med. 2010;39:696–700.

[67] Phillips S, Pemberton JH. Acute megacolon. In: Sleisenger MH, Fordtran JS, editors. Gastrointestinal diseases: pathophysiology, diagnosis, management. Philadelphia: WB Sanders Co; 1998. p. 1817–1818.

[68] Sanders MD, Kimmel MB. Systematic review: acute colonic pseudo-obstruction. Aliment Pharmacol Ther. 2005;22:917–925.

[69] De Giorgio R, Barbara G, Stanghellini V et al. Review article: the pharmacological treatment of acute colonic pseudo-obstruction. Aliment Pharmacol Ther. 2001;15:1717–1727.

[70] Tenofsky PL, Beamer L, Smith RS. Ogilvie syndrome as a postoperative complication. Arch Surg. 2000;135:682–687.

[71] Geller A, Petersen PT, Gostout CJ. Endoscopic decompression for acute colonic pseudo-obstruction. Gastrointest Endosc. 1996;44:144–150.

[72] Feldstein AE, Miller SM, El-Youssef M et al. Chronic intestinal pseudo-obstruction associated with altered interstitial cells of Cajal network. J Pediatr Gastroenterol Nutr. 2003;36:492–497.

[73] Schuffler MD, Deitch EA. Chronic idiopathic intestinal pseudo-obstruction. A surgical approach. Am Surg. 1980;192:752.

Chapter 3

Risk Factors and Predictive Models for Conversion of Laparoscopic Cholecystectomy to Open Surgery, and Surgical Quality Outcome Measures

Andrei M. Beliaev and Michael Booth

Additional information is available at the end of the chapter

http://dx.doi.org/10.5772/63648

Abstract

Background: Laparoscopic cholecystectomy is the preferred surgical operation for symptomatic gallstone disease. Conversion of laparoscopic cholecystectomy to open surgery is used to prevent intra-abdominal organ injury, for open common bile duct exploration and to repair intra-abdominal organ injury.

Objective: The objective of this chapter is to review risk factors and predictive models for conversion of laparoscopic cholecystectomy to open surgery, and surgical quality outcome measures.

Methods: A narrative literature review using Pubmed, Medline, Cochrane library databases and Google search engine is described.

Results: From the literature review, patient- and surgeon-related risk factors and predictive models for conversion of laparoscopic cholecystectomy to open surgery were identified. Patient-dependent risk factors included preoperative and intraoperative variables. Current conversion of laparoscopic cholecystectomy to open surgery predictive models use only patient-dependent risk factors and were not tested on an independent sample of patients. Surgical quality outcome measures incorporate an association between conversion and intra-abdominal organ injury that demonstrates that conversion was used as an emergency strategy to repair injuries rather than a safety measure.

Conclusion: Conversion of laparoscopic cholecystectomy to open surgery risk stratification based on patient- and surgeon-dependent variables may allow a better management of the patient to keep conversion at low rates and to maintain benefits of minimally invasive surgery.

Keywords: laparoscopic cholecystectomy, conversion to open surgery, risk factors, predictive models, intra-abdominal organ injury, surgical quality indicators

---

1. Introduction

The prevalence of cholelithiasis in an adult Western population is between 15 and 20% [1, 2]. In the United States, an estimated 11.8 million people aged between 20 and 74 years have gallbladder (GB) stones [3]. Yearly approximately 1–2% of patients with silent gallstones develop symptoms and require treatment (**Figure 1**) [4–6]. Acute cholecystitis (AC) accounts for 20% of patients presented to hospital with right upper quadrant pain, which in patients with significant co-morbidities and in the elderly is associated with 2–3% mortality [5, 7, 8]. In the United States, in 2009, cholecystitis was the underlying cause of death in 2009 patients and a contributing cause of death in 3295 patients accounting for a mortality crude rate of 0.7 per 100,000 patients [9]. In the same country, GB disease is one of the most common inpatient diagnosis that accounts for more than 260,000 hospital admissions and annual health care provider expenditure exceeding $3.03 billion [9].

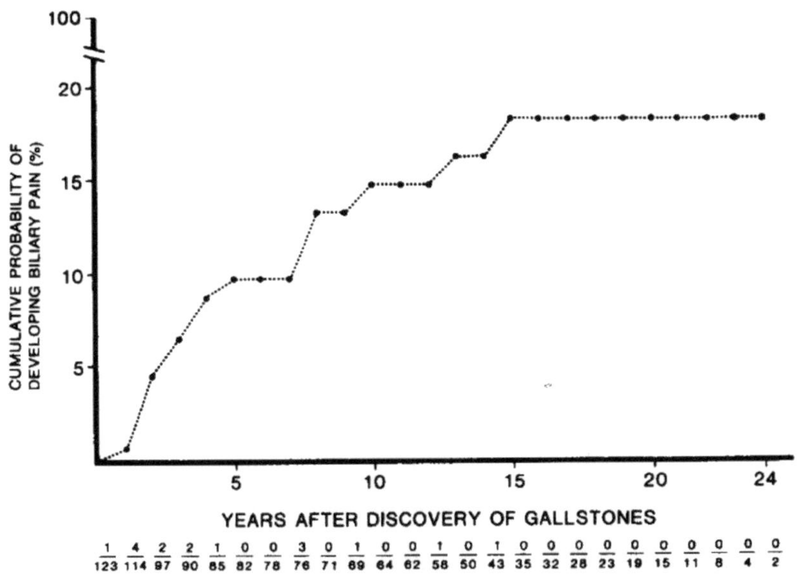

Figure 1. Life-table analysis of the outcome of silent gallstone disease. The fractions along the abscissa show the number of people developing biliary pain over the number at risk (adapted from Gracie and Ransohoff [4]).

Laparoscopic cholecystectomy (LC) is considered as the "gold standard" surgical technique for treatment of GB disease [10]. Conversion of LC to open surgery (CTO) is used to prevent intra-abdominal organ injury (IOI), for common bile duct (CBD) exploration and to repair IOI.

The aim of this chapter is to review risk factors and predictive models for CTO, and surgical quality outcome measures.

2. Laparoscopic cholecystectomy

LC is the minimally invasive surgical operation that was introduced in clinical practice by Erich Muehe of Boeblingen, Germany, in 1985 [11]. LC can be performed with the conventional four-port or three-port technique.

Compared to the conventional open cholecystectomy (OC), LC has decreased post-operative pain, decreased respiratory function dysfunction, reduced post-operative ileus, earlier oral fluid and food intake, better cosmesis, reduced patient's hospital stay, fastened post-operative recovery and lowered morbidity and mortality [12–14].

A meta-analysis comparing LC with the small-incision OC (the length of incision of less than 8 cm) demonstrated that both techniques had similar rates of mortality; intraoperative, minor and severe post-operative complications (without bile duct injuries, BDI); BDI; total complications; and post-operative convalescence [15]. A subgroup analysis of high-quality trials showed a shorter operative time for the small-incision OC than LC (weighted mean difference, random effects 16.4 min, 95% CI: 8.9–23.8 min) [15]. Compared with the small-incision OC, the self-reported quality of life up to 30 days after LC is higher; 2326 (95% CI: 2187–2391) and 2411 (95% CI: 2334–2502), respectively, $P = 0.03$ [16].

Main disadvantages of LC compared to the conventional OC and small-incision OC are a lack of a three-dimensional view, narrow field of laparoscopic vision, inconvenience with liver retraction, insufficient tactile sensations due to manipulation with long laparoscopic instruments and difficulties with instruments placement and manoeuvring [17–19].

Another significant limitation of LC is an increased risk of IOI, including bile duct injury (BDI) [20, 21]. In the United States, approximately 750,000 LCs are performed annually [22]. With the incidence of major BDI during LC fluctuating between 0.4 and 2%, it is expected that 3000 to 15,000 patients will suffer from iatrogenic BDI [21, 23, 24]. Major BDI is associated with significant morbidity, mortality and socioeconomic burden [21].

2.1. Indications for conversion of LC to open surgery

The primary indication for CTO is to prevent IOI. CTO can also be used for CBD exploration, to repair cholecysto-intestinal fistula and to perform an extended OC in patients with gallbladder cancer. In addition, CTO is performed to control haemorrhage and repair single or multiple IOI [25, 26].

Compared to LC, CTO is associated with an increased morbidity and mortality. A clinical audit of 7242 LCs for AC performed in the United States between 2005 and 2011 showed that compared to the LC group, patients who underwent CTO had higher rates of surgical site infection (1.8 versus 9.2%, $P < 0.0001$), operations for complications (1.4 versus 3.4%, $P = 0.001$), serious morbidity (3.8 versus 14.9%, $P < 0.0001$), overall morbidity (6.0 versus 21.8%, $P < 0.0001$) and mortality (0.5 versus 2.3%, $P < 0.0001$) [18]. In addition, the CTO group of patients had a longer mean operation time (122.1 ± 51.0 min versus 80.0 ± 42.6 min, $P < 0.0001$) as well as the length of hospital stay (8.6 ± 13.0 days versus 3.4 ± 6.7 days, $P < 0.0001$) than LC patients [18].

2.2. Risk factors for conversion of LC to open surgery

As high rate of CTO and IOI can diminish clinical benefits and cost-effectiveness of LC, identification of preoperative and intraoperative patient-dependent and surgeon-related risk factors for CTO can be used for development of risk stratification models and refinement of the management. This will keep CTO at low rates and maintain benefits of minimally invasive GB surgery.

2.2.1. Preoperative patient-related risk factors

Preoperative patient-related risk factors for CTO have been extensively investigated and identified. In previous studies, the advanced age has been shown to be a risk factor for CTO [25, 27, 28]. In a meta-analysis, Yang et al. demonstrated that age >65 years is associated with a twofold increase in CTO rate (odds ratio (OR) = 1.8; 95% confidence interval (CI): 1.4–2.5; $P < 0.0001$) (**Table 1**) [29]. These findings can be explained by a higher proportion of severe AC, GB cancer, choledocholithiasis and previous abdominal operations among the older patients compared to their younger counterparts [28, 30].

Preoperative patient-related risk factors for CTO	OR	95% CI	*P* value	References
Advanced age (>65 years)	1.8	1.4–2.5	<0.0001	[29]
Male	2.8	1.1–6.6	0.037	[32]
Clinical diagnosis of AC	8	6.1–10.5	<0.00005	[35]
Duration of AC >72 h	3.1	1.2–7.7	0.0072	[37]
Repeated attacks of AC, ≥2	7.9	1.5–76.8	<0.0052	[41]
Diabetes mellitus	2.5	1.3–4.4	0.003	[43]
Obesity, BMI >30 kg/m^2	7.6	4.1–14	<0.001	[52]
Previous upper abdominal surgery	20.4	2.4–927.4	0.0007	[50]
Post-ERC/ES, ≥16 weeks	3	1.2–7.4	0.009	[57]
WCC ≥ 11 × 10^9/L	4	2.5–6.1	<0.00005	[25]
Elevated CRP, 10 mg/L	1.05	1.01–1.09	0.014	[37]
Elevated total bilirubin	6.5	4.1–10.2	<0.00005	[64]
Alkaline phosphatase (>135 U/L)	7	3.6–14	<0.00001	[52]
Gallbladder wall thickness, mm	2	1.7–2.3	<0.00005	[52]
Pericholecystic fluid on US	26	5.0–166.1	<0.00005	[41]
ASA score >2	2.5	1.3–4.6	0.004	[66]

Abbreviations: CTO, conversion of laparoscopic cholecystectomy to open surgery; OR, odds ratio; CI, confidence interval; AC, acute cholecystitis; BMI, body mass index; ERC/ES, endoscopic retrograde cholangiography with endoscopic sphincterotomy; WCC, white cell count; CRP, C-reactive protein; U, units; L, litre; ASA, American Society of Anaesthesiologist; US, trans-abdominal ultrasound.

Table 1. Preoperative patient-related risk factors for conversion of laparoscopic cholecystectomy to open surgery.

A. Local signs of inflammation, etc.:
(1) Murphy's sign, (2) RUQ mass/pain/tenderness
B. Systemic signs of inflammation, etc.:
(1) Fever, (2) raised WCC, (3) elevated CRP
C. Imaging findings: imaging findings characteristic of acute cholecystitis
(1) Trans-abdominal ultrasound findings:
Positive sonographic Murphy sign (ultrasound transducer elicited tenderness on gentle pressure over the gallbladder
Thickened gallbladder wall (>4 mm, provided there is no congestive heart failure, chronic liver disease and ascites)
Marked distension of the gallbladder (long axis diameter >80 mm, short axis diameter >40 mm)
Gallstone impacted in Hartman's pouch; biliary sludge, pericholecystic fluid collection
Sonolucent halo in the gallbladder wall
(2) CT findings:
Gallbladder distension
Gallbladder subserosal oedema
Gallbladder wall thickening
Pericholecystic stranding, fluid collection
(3) Magnetic resonance imaging findings:
Cystic duct stone
Intraluminal sludge
Pericholecystic high signal
Gallbladder distension
Gallbladder wall thickening, abnormal signal intensity and oedematous stratification
(4) Tc-HIDA scan findings:
Non-visualized gallbladder within 1 h
"Rim sign" (increased pericholecystic hepatic radioactivity)
Suspected diagnosis: One item in A + one item in B
Definite diagnosis: One item in A + one item in B + C

Note: acute hepatitis, other acute abdominal diseases, and chronic cholecystitis should be excluded.
Abbreviations: RUQ, right upper abdominal quadrant; CRP, C-reactive protein; WCC, white cell count; US, ultrasound; MRI, magnetic resonance imaging; CT, computed tomography; Tc-HIDA scan, 99mTc-hepatic iminodiacetic acid cholescintigraphy.

Table 2. The 2013 Tokyo guidelines diagnostic criteria for acute cholecystitis (modified from Yokoe et al. [34]).

Male gender is a well-recognized risk factor for difficult LC and CTO [18, 25, 28, 29]. Males have more prominent adhesions between the GB and the omentum and surrounding internal organs, have a higher proportion of severe forms of AC on histological examination of the GB, have a higher CTO rate and require a longer operation time [31]. Two-stage LC male patients have a three times higher rate of CTO (OR = 2.8; 95% CI: 1.1–6.6, $P = 0.037$) than females [32]. This might be due to men's reluctance to seek medical and surgical help, and their late hospital presentations after several repeated attacks of AC [31].

Patients with the clinical diagnosis of AC and higher severity grades of AC carry more chances of CTO [25, 33, 34]. Diagnostic criteria for AC are presented in **Table 2** [34]. AC patients have eight times higher risk of CTO than patients with uncomplicated gallstone disease (OR = 8.01; 95% CI: 6.1–10.5; $P < 0.00005$) [35]. Severity grades of AC, as defined by the 2013 Tokyo Guidelines, are associated with an increased rate of CTO [36, 37]. The 2013 Tokyo Guidelines for severity grades of AC are shown in **Table 3** [34]. Severe AC makes LC technically more difficult, because AC is accompanied by extensive adhesions around GB and weakness of the GB wall, which preclude its retraction with laparoscopic forceps and cause GB perforation and spillage of infected bile and gallstones into the peritoneal cavity [32].

Grade I (mild) acute cholecystitis
Does not meet the criteria of "grade III" or "grade II" acute cholecystitis. Grade I can also be defined as acute cholecystitis in a healthy patient with no organ dysfunction and mild inflammatory changes in the gallbladder, making cholecystectomy a safe and low-risk operative procedure
Moderate (grade II) acute cholecystitis
Grade II (moderate) acute cholecystitis
Associated with any one of the following conditions:
1. Elevated white cell count (>18,000/mm^3)
2. Palpable tender mass in the right upper quadrant
3. Duration of complaints > 72 h
4. Marked local inflammation (gangrenous cholecystitis, pericholecystic abscess, hepatic abscess, biliary peritonitis, emphysematous cholecystitis)
Grade III (severe) acute cholecystitis
Associated with dysfunction of any one of the following organs/systems:
1. Cardiovascular dysfunction (hypotension requiring treatment with dopamine ≥5 mcg/kg/min, or any dose of norepinephrine)
2. Neurological dysfunction (decreased level of consciousness)
3. Respiratory dysfunction (PaO_2/FiO_2 ratio <300)
4. Renal dysfunction (oliguria, creatinine >2.0 mg/dL)
5. Hepatic dysfunction (PT-INR >1.5)
6. Haematological dysfunction (platelet count <100,000/mm^3)

Table 3. The 2013 Tokyo guidelines severity grading for acute cholecystitis (adapted from Yokoe et al. [34]).

The longer the duration of untreated AC, the greater is the risk for CTO [27]. Asai et al. showed that 12 of 29 (41.4%) patients in the CTO group and 36 of 196 (18.4%) patients in LC group had symptoms of AC for longer than 72 h ($P = 0.0004$) [37]. Therefore, untreated AC lasting more than 2 days increases the risk for CTO by three times (OR 3.1; 95% CI: 1.2–7.7; $P = 0.0072$).

Repeated attacks of AC are associated with difficult LC and CTO [38–40]. When compared to AC patients with less than two previous episodes, patients with at least two past attacks of AC have an eightfold increase in the difficulty of LC (OR = 7.9; 95% CI: 3.4–18.2; $P < 0.00005$) and the rate of CTO (OR = 7.9; 95% CI: 1.5–76.8; $P = 0.0052$) [41]. Compared to patients with one previous attack of AC, having at least three attacks of AC escalates LC difficulty by a factor of 28 (OR = 28.3; 95% CI: 7.4–127.6; $P < 0.00005$) and increases the rate of CTO a 14-fold (OR = 14.1; 95% CI: 2.1–153.2; $P = 0.0021$) [41].

Diabetes mellitus (DM) has been consistently shown to be associated with CTO [18, 25, 42]. Diabetics undergoing LC have a 2.5 times higher risk for CTO than nondiabetic patients (OR = 2.5; 95% CI: 1.3–4.4, $P = 0.003$) [43]. This might be because diabetic patients have a threefold greater risk for the development of AC than non-diabetics (OR 2.7; 95% CI: 1.8–4.2; $P < 0.00005$) [44]. Also, diabetics, especially if they are on insulin, have an 85% increased risk of preoperative GB perforation (adjusted OR = 1.85; 95% CI: 1.38–2.48; $P < 0.001$) [45]. Poor glycaemic control and presence of diabetic microagiopathy and autonomic neuropathy, as well as frequent bactibilia, are important conditions that predispose diabetics to advanced forms of AC and infective complications [40, 46–49].

Obesity (body mass index (BMI) > 30 kg/m^2) is not only a risk factor for CTO but also associated with major BDI [18, 28, 50, 51]. Obese patients undergoing LC have an eightfold higher risk of CTO than non-obese patients (OR = 7.6; 95% CI: 4.1–14; $P < 0.001$) [52]. Compared to the non-obese patients, class I and class II–III obese patients have a two- and threefold increase in the risk of CTO (OR = 1.8; 95% CI: 1.1–2.8; $P = 0.0105$) and (OR = 2.7; 95% CI: 1.5–4.6; $P = 0.0006$), respectively [53].

Previous surgery above the umbilicus is a risk factor for CTO [52, 54]. In Lee's study, 7 (17%) of 41 patients from the CTO group and 1 (1%) of 100 patients from the LC group had a history of previous upper abdominal surgery [50]. This estimates the risk for CTO for patients with the past history of upper abdominal surgery 20 times higher than for those without previous surgery above the umbilicus (OR = 20.4, 95% CI: 2.4–927.4; $P = 0.0007$).

The risk of CTO is also higher in patients following endoscopic retrograde cholangiography with sphincterotomy (ERC/ES) for CBD stone clearance [54–56]. A two-stage LC after 15 weeks following ERC/ES increases the rate of CTO three times (RR = 2.7, 95% CI: 1.4–5.5, $P = 0.004$) and major BDI 10-fold (RR = 10.2, 95% CI: 1.1–95.7, $P = 0.043$) [57]. Boerma et al. compared the two-stage LC conducted within 6 weeks after ERC with that performed after 6 weeks and found that the latter was more technically demanding and associated with a threefold increase in the CTO rate (RR = 2.7, 95% CI: 1.3–3.4, $P = 0.01$) [58]. An association between preoperative ERC/ES and difficult LC can be explained by bactibilia-related inflammation of bile ducts with desmoplastic changes around the Calot's triangle and shrinking of the GB [59, 60].

Thickened gallbladder wall on ultrasound (US) of the upper abdomen is associated with CTO [25, 28]. The risk of CTO doubles with every millimetre increase in gallbladder wall thickness (OR = 2; 95% CI: 1.7–2.3; $P < 0.001$) [52]. Patients with GB wall thickness >5 mm on trans-abdominal US have a 16 times higher risk of CTO than those with GB wall thickness 3–5 mm (OR = 16.3; 95% CI: 8.1–33.3; $P < 0.00005$) [35]. GB wall thickness >4 mm on US is not only a radiological marker for AC but also associated with greater operational difficulty [40, 61].

The presence of pericholecystic fluid on imaging of the abdomen increases the risk of CTO by 26 times (OR = 26; 95% CI: 5.0–166.1; $P < 0.00005$) [41]. This radiological sign has the sensitivity of 70% in predicting CTO, the specificity of 92%, the positive predictive value of 33% and the negative predictive value of 98% [41].

An elevated white cell count (WCC) is a predictor of CTO [28]. Compared to the LC group, the CTO group had a higher proportion of patients with leucocytosis, defined as WCC ≥ 11 × 10^9/L, 161 (12.7%) of 1265 patients versus 41 (36.6%) of 112 patients, respectively, $P < 0.001$ [25]. This estimates a fourfold higher risk of CTO among patients with WCC ≥ 11 × 10^9/L (OR = 4.0; 95% CI: 2.5–6.1) compared with leucopenic and patients with normal WCC (WCC ≤ 11 × 10^9/L), $P < 0.00005$. In another study, Nidoni et al. showed that the sensitivity of WCC ≥ 11 ×10^9/L in predicting CTO is 80%, the specificity 83.5%, the positive and negative predictive values 22.2 and 98.6%, respectively [41].

Histopathology of acute cholecystitis	WCC cut-off (95% CI)	CRP cut-off (95% CI)	AUC of WCC (95% CI)	AUC of CRP (95% CI)	*P* value
Overall AC	9.15 (8.7–9.6)	30.5 (10.2–50.8)	0.83 (0.79–0.87)	0.94 (0.92–0.97)	<0.00005
Mild AC	9.01 (8.7–9.32)	26.5 (13.6–39.4)	0.79 (0.74–0.84)	0.93 (0.9–0.95)	<0.00005
Moderate-severe AC	11.05 (10.22–11.88)	67 (61.9–72.1)	0.92 (0.88–0.97)	0.99 (0.97–1.0)	0.0093
Acute on chronic cholecystitis	9.15 (8.81–9.49)	26.5 (15.72–37.28)	0.72 (0.65–0.79)	0.87 (0.82–0.92)	0.0004
Acute edematous cholecystitis	9.05 (8.29–9.81)	30.5 (3.34–51.68)	0.78 (0.69–0.87)	0.93 (0.87–0.99)	0.0001
Acute necrotizing cholecystitis	9.05 (6.97–11.12)	57.5 (34.74–80.26)	0.89 (0.83–0.95)	0.97 (0.94–1.0)	0.0149
Acute suppurative cholecystitis	9.15 (7.96–10.34)	92 (76.43–111.57)	0.82 (0.67–0.97)	1.0 (1.0–1.0)	0.0189
Acute gangrenous cholecystitis	11.65 (10.63–12.67)	67 (61.78–72.22)	0.93 (0.89–0.98)	0.99 (0.97–1.0)	0.0375
Pericholecystic abscess/ gallbladder perforation	9.15 (7.82–10.48)	86 (66.28–105.72)	0.89 (0.76–1.0)	1.0 (1.0–1.0)	0.0852

Abbreviations: CRP, C-reactive protein; WCC, white cell count; AC, acute cholecystitis; AUC, the area under receiver operating characteristic curve.

Table 4. Cut-off values and areas under receiver operating characteristic curve of CRP and WCC in acute cholecystitis (adapted from Beliaev et al. [63]).

An elevated C-reactive protein (CRP) level also predicts CTO [62]. Every 10 mg/L increase in CRP concentration, the rate of CTO increases by 5% (OR = 1.05; 95% CI: 1.01–1.09; $P = 0.014$) [37]. The cut-off point of CRP > 115 mg/L predicts CTO with the sensitivity of 79% and specificity of 57%. CRP as a predictor of CTO has the area under receiver operating characteristic curve (AUC) of 67% [37]. An association between CTO and CRP concentration can be explained by severity of AC. The cut-off point of CRP concentration increases with more advanced histological forms of AC and its severity grades (**Table 4**) [63].

Deranged liver function tests predict CTO [28, 64]. Patients with elevated concentrations of total bilirubin and alkaline phosphatase (>135 U/L) have seven times higher risk of CTO, OR = 6.5 (95% CI: 4.1–10.2; $P < 0.00005$) and OR = 7.0 (95% CI: 3.6–14; $P < 0.00001$), respectively [25, 52]. Elevated levels of total bilirubin and alkaline phosphatase are both independently associated with choledocholithiasis [65]. Open CBD exploration is one of the reasons for CTO.

An increasing ASA score has been shown in multiple studies to be an independent risk factor for CTO [25, 27, 28, 52, 62, 66]. Patients with ASA score of 3 have 2.5 times odds of CTO (OR = 2.5; 95% CI: 1.3–4.6) than those with ASA score of 1 ($P = 0.004$) [66].

2.2.2. *Intraoperative patient-related risk factors*

To prevent IOI during LC, when the surgeon encounters dense intra-abdominal adhesions, extensive inflammatory changes around the gallbladder, haemorrhage, inability to grasp and retract a friable gallbladder with forceps, CTO is advised [67].

Severe intra-abdominal adhesions make laparoscopic dissection very difficult and are associated with a fivefold increase in CTO risk (OR = 5.2; 95% CI: 1.9–14.4; $P = 0.002$) [32]. Some authors report their institutional policy of avoidance of difficult dissections during LC and making a decision of CTO if there is a lack of dissection progress for 15–30 min [27].

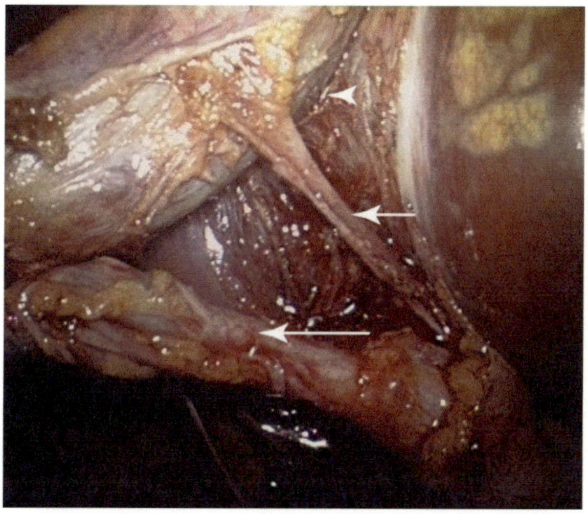

Figure 2. Critical view of safety. The arrowhead shows detachment of the lowest part of the gallbladder from the gallbladder bed, the smaller arrow depicts the cystic artery and the larger arrow points at the cystic duct.

Intense inflammatory infiltrate in the Calot's triangle makes identification of the cystic duct and cystic artery very challenging predisposing patients to iatrogenic BDI and uncontrollable bleeding [32, 35]. To prevent BDI, CTO is directed when one of three fundamentals of the critical view of safety cannot be ascertained [30, 68]. These essentials include the clearance of the Calot's triangle from adipose and fibrous tissue, detachment of the lowest part of the gallbladder from the GB bed and identification of the cystic duct and cystic artery going into the gallbladder (**Figure 2**) [69]. Alternatively, when the surgeon encounters severe inflammatory or desmoplastic reaction in the Calot's triangle laparoscopic subtotal cholecystectomy can be performed [70–72].

Unclear biliary anatomy is another reason for CTO [20]. Instead, intraoperative cholangiography (IOC) can be used to prevent misidentification of the cystic duct and prevent BDI [73, 74]. Failure of the contrast to opacify the common hepatic duct and the right and left hepatic ducts would signal the surgeon that the CBD, not the cystic duct, has been cannulated [74]. The use of IOC is associated with a 62% reduction in CTO rate (OR = 0.38, 95% CI: 0.17–0.94; $P = 0.04$) [75]. If IOC does not facilitate unmistakeable biliary ducts recognition, then CTO is indicated [74].

Intraoperative patient-related risk factors for CTO
Adhesions caused by previous upper abdominal operations
Adhesions in the upper abdomen caused by severe pericholecystic tissue inflammation
Enlarged fatty liver (steatohepatitis) restricting access and inability to elevate gallbladder to dissect Calot's triangle
Intra-hepatic gallbladder
Necrotic gallbladder wall
Thickened sclerotic gallbladder wall/porcelain gallbladder
Gallbladder perforation with biliary peritonitis
Large gallbladder stone impacted in Hartman's pouch/Mirizzi syndrome
Fibrosis of tissue in Calot's triangle
Severe inflammation in Calot's triangle
Uncontrollable bleeding from cystic artery, hepatic artery, gallbladder bed
Cholecysto-intestinal fistula
Unclear biliary anatomy
Choledocholithiasis requiring open CBD exploration
Suspicion of gallbladder cancer
Intra-abdominal organs injury
Intolerance of intraperitoneal carbon dioxide insufflation

Abbreviations: CTO, conversion of laparoscopic cholecystectomy to open surgery; CBD, common bile duct.

Table 5. Intraoperative patient-related risk factors that may require conversion of laparoscopic cholecystectomy to open surgery.

CTO is performed when open CBD exploration and stone clearance is required provided CBD stones cannot be removed laparoscopically or post-operatively by ERC/ES [20, 76, 77]. Furthermore, CTO is advised for an open repair of intraoperatively diagnosed IOI [20, 25]. Infrequently, CTO is necessary when the patient is not able to tolerate 12 mm Hg intraperitoneal carbon dioxide insufflation pressure and develops premature ventricular beats and bradycardia with hypotension [20].

Intraoperative patient-related risk factors that may require conversion of laparoscopic cholecystectomy to open surgery are presented in **Table 5.**

2.2.3. Surgeon-related risk factors

Surgeon's knowledge, laparoscopic fellowship training, operative experience and skills in laparoscopic surgery play an important role in timely recognition of the need for CTO and are important predictors for CTO [49, 74, 75, 78]. Surgical registrars (postgraduate year 4–5) have a twofold higher rate of CTO (OR = 1.7; 95% CI: 1.1–2.5; $P = 0.0067$) than surgical consultants [25]. Compared to general surgical registrars without fellowship training, completion of the surgical fellowship program is associated with 92% reduction in the rate of CTO (OR = 0.08; 95% CI: 0.02–0.32, $P < 0.0001$) [79].

Importantly, there is statistically significant inverse correlation between surgeons' LC volume and the rate of CTO ($P = 0.03$) [80]. The surgeons with more than 5 years of experience in independent practice, who performed at least 100 LC or more than 75 cases annually are considered to be experts, and the surgeons with personal records of less than 100 LC as the first surgeons to be non-experts [81, 82]. In addition, surgeon's specialization influences the incidence of CTO. The expertise of upper gastrointestinal (UGI) surgeons is recognized to be the standard in LC against which the other surgeons' capability can be measured. Compared to the UGI surgeons, non-UGI surgeons have a two times higher incidence of CTO (OR = 2.1; 95% CI: 1.1–3.7; $P = 0.0122$) [80].

2.3. Predictive models for conversion of LC to open surgery

Few predictive models have been developed to help the surgeon make an early CTO decision. Lipman et al. found that variables such as male gender, WCC $\geq 11 \times 10^9$/L, low albumin, pericholecystic fluid on US, the presence of diabetes mellitus and elevated total bilirubin independently predict CTO. These risk factors were included into the model which has the AUC of 83%. The authors showed that if none of these risk factors were present, the risk of conversion is 2%, but when six risk factors were present, the risk of conversion escalated to 90% [25].

Kama et al. presented a CTO risk scoring model consisting of a constant (-20) and six variables with their coefficients, age ≥60 years (coefficient of 5), male gender (11), previous upper abdominal surgery (8), abdominal tenderness (9), thickness of gallbladder wall >4 mm on US (13) and the clinical diagnosis of AC (15) [83]. The final risk score for CTO (RSCLO) is the sum of the constant and coefficients of the risk factors that are present in an individual patient. The

RSCLO can take a value between −20 and 41. An operation with RSCLO exceeding −3 is considered difficult [84].

Goonawardena et al. proposed a CTO prediction model that is constructed on five independent variables, previous upper abdominal surgery, obesity (BMI > 30 kg/m^2) and the presence of choledocholithiasis, impacted stone at the Hartmann's pouch and GB wall thickening on the trans-abdominal US [52].

Sugrue et al. developed an intraoperative 10-point scoring system for an assessment of the difficulty in LC [85]. A score of <2 indicates mild degree difficulty, 2–4 moderate, 5–7 severe and 8–10 the extreme difficulty of LC [85].

These predictive models have limitations. They have not been tested on an independent sample. Therefore, their real-life predictive ability is unknown. In addition, these models excluded surgeon-related risk factors. Thus, it is difficult to tailor management of high-risk for CTO patients according to an available hepato-biliary expertise.

3. Outcomes and quality indicators in laparoscopic cholecystectomy

Time to operation theatre (*TTO*) is the period between hospital admission and the start of operation. TTO is correlated with the length of the index hospital admission and associated with an increased expenditure for health care provider. Fry et al. showed that the length of preoperative hospitalization exceeding 3 days (96 h) incurs an added cost of 2011 US$ 7584 [86].

The CTO rate is the proportion of cases of LC converted to open surgery to the total number of intended LC. Mueller et al. consider CTO as a quality variable, because CTO is associated with a worse outcome [87]. Other authors do not regard CTO as a complication, but rather as a "sign of experience" or "mature judgment" to prevent IOI [20, 28]. We classify all CTO into three groups: (1) the safety CTO when conversion is performed to prevent IOI; (2) conversion of LC to extended surgery is implemented for an open CBD exploration, for closure of cholecysto-intestinal fistula, or for an extended OC in case of GB cancer; and (3) the emergency CTO is performed to stop bleeding or repair IOI detected intraoperatively. In this view, safety CTO and extended surgery CTO are not complications, but carefully thought-out surgical strategies.

Laparoscopic BDI rate is the proportion of injury to bile ducts that occurred during LC to the total number of LCs. Commonly, BDIs are specified according to the Strasberg's classification [88].

IOI rate is the proportion of iatrogenic injury to one or more intra-abdominal organs, including the liver, bile ducts, small and large bowel, stomach, spleen, pancreas, mesentery and vascular injury accompanied with extensive haemorrhage to the total number of cholecystectomies.

An association between CTO and IOI is a surgical quality indicator that shows that CTO is used predominantly as an emergency surgical strategy to control haemorrhage and repair IOI diagnosed intraoperatively [89].

Procedures or operations performed for treatment of complications are procedures performed for complications during the index hospital admission and readmissions.

Severity of post-operative complications can be graded using the Dindo-Clavien classification [90]. This classification does not specify the hospital admission during which they developed. We suggest using the Dindo-Clavien classification to grade post-operative complications that arose during the index hospital admission.

The length of stay (*LOS*) is the duration of the index hospital admission.

Readmission within 30 or 90 days from the index hospital discharge is the readmission to any acute care hospital with a condition that could be considered an outcome of the procedure or operation [86]. To define readmissions period, some authors use a 30-day period after the index hospital admission discharge, the others a 90-day period [86, 91, 92]. We think that the 90-day post-index hospital stay readmission period is more meaningful, because it is more likely to capture an adverse event due to a retained CBD stone rather than a 30-day period.

The post-operative length of stay (LOS) below 2 days (72 *h*) *with no hospital readmission* is an indicator of an uncomplicated cholecystectomy [93].

The prolonged post-operative LOS exceeding 3 days (96 *h*) is an indicator of protracted admission after LC.

The total length of hospital stay includes the length of the index hospital admission and duration of readmissions within 90-day post-index hospital stay discharge.

Thirty-day or 90-day postdischarge death is the death that occurs within 30 days or 90 days from either the index hospital admission or hospital readmission discharge.

Patient-reported outcome measures including generic (the Short Form 36 (SF-36) Health Survey, Nottingham Health Profile), preference-based (European Quality of Life Questionnaire, EQ-5D) and condition-specific instruments (Otago Gallstones Condition-Specific Questionnaire, Gastrointestinal Quality of Life Index, Abdominal Surgery Impact Scale and Gallstone Impact Checklist) as well as economic evaluations (cost–minimization analysis, cost–consequence analysis, cost–effectiveness analysis, cost–utility analysis and cost–benefit analysis) can also be used as outcome measures.

4. Conclusion

LC is the treatment of choice for symptomatic GB disease, which in some patients requires CTO. CTO risk stratification based on patient- and surgeon-dependent variables may allow a better patient's management to keep CTO at low rates and maintain benefits of minimally invasive GB surgery. The absence of an association between CTO and IOI is an important surgical safety indicator that demonstrates that CTO is used as a safety strategy rather than an emergency measure to repair iatrogenic IOI and control haemorrhage.

Author details

Andrei M. Beliaev[1*] and Michael Booth[2]

*Address all correspondence to: Andrei.Belyaev@adhb.govt.nz

1 Auckland City Hospital, Auckland, New Zealand

2 North Shore Hospital, Auckland, New Zealand

References

[1] Glambek I, Kvaale G, Arnesjo B, Soreide O. Prevalence of gallstones in a Norwegian population. Scand J Gastroenterol. [Research Support, Non-U.S. Gov't]. 1987 Nov;22(9): 1089–94.

[2] Muhrbeck O, Ahlberg J. Prevalence of gallstone disease in a Swedish population. Scand J Gastroenterol. [Research Support, Non-U.S. Gov't]. 1995 Nov;30(11):1125–8.

[3] Everhart JE, Khare M, Hill M, Maurer KR. Prevalence and ethnic differences in gallbladder disease in the United States. Gastroenterology. 1999 Sep;117(3):632–9.

[4] Gracie WA, Ransohoff DF. The natural history of silent gallstones: the innocent gallstone is not a myth. N Engl J Med. 1982 Sep 23;307(13):798–800.

[5] Halldestam I, Enell EL, Kullman E, Borch K. Development of symptoms and complications in individuals with asymptomatic gallstones. Br J Surg. 2004 Jun;91(6):734–8.

[6] Friedman GD. Natural history of asymptomatic and symptomatic gallstones. Am J Surg. [Research Support, U.S. Gov't, P.H.S.Review]. 1993 Apr;165(4):399–404.

[7] Papadakis M, Ambe PC, Zirngibl H. Critically ill patients with acute cholecystitis are at increased risk for extensive gallbladder inflammation. World J Emerg Surg. 2015;10:59.

[8] Haltmeier T, Benjamin E, Inaba K, Lam L, Demetriades D. Early versus delayed same-admission laparoscopic cholecystectomy for acute cholecystitis in elderly patients with comorbidities. J Trauma Acute Care Surg. 2015 Apr;78(4):801–7.

[9] Peery AF, Dellon ES, Lund J, Crockett SD, McGowan CE, Bulsiewicz WJ, et al. Burden of gastrointestinal disease in the United States: 2012 update. Gastroenterology. [Research Support, N.I.H., Extramural Research Support, Non-U.S. Gov't]. 2012 Nov; 143(5):1179–87 e1–3.

[10] Agresta F, Campanile FC, Vettoretto N, Silecchia G, Bergamini C, Maida P, et al. Laparoscopic cholecystectomy: consensus conference-based guidelines. Langenbecks Arch Surg. [Review]. 2015 May;400(4):429–53.

[11] Reynolds W, Jr. The first laparoscopic cholecystectomy. Jsls. [Biography Historical Article Portraits]. 2001 Jan–Mar;5(1):89–94.

[12] Csikesz N, Ricciardi R, Tseng JF, Shah SA. Current status of surgical management of acute cholecystitis in the United States. World J Surg. [Comparative Study Multicenter Study Research Support, Non-U.S. Gov't]. 2008 Oct;32(10):2230–6.

[13] Keus F, de Jong JA, Gooszen HG, van Laarhoven CJ. Laparoscopic versus open cholecystectomy for patients with symptomatic cholecystolithiasis. Cochrane Database Syst Rev. [Meta-Analysis Research Support, Non-U.S. Gov't Review]. 2006(4):CD006231.

[14] Bablekos GD, Michaelides SA, Analitis A, Charalabopoulos KA. Effects of laparoscopic cholecystectomy on lung function: a systematic review. World J Gastroenterol. [Meta-Analysis Review]. 2014 Dec 14;20(46):17603–17.

[15] Keus F, Gooszen HG, Van Laarhoven CJ. Systematic review: open, small-incision or laparoscopic cholecystectomy for symptomatic cholecystolithiasis. Aliment Pharmacol Ther. [Review]. 2009 Feb 15;29(4):359–78.

[16] Rosenmuller MH, Thoren Ornberg M, Myrnas T, Lundberg O, Nilsson E, Haapamaki MM. Expertise-based randomized clinical trial of laparoscopic versus small-incision open cholecystectomy. Br J Surg. [Comparative Study Randomized Controlled Trial Research Support, Non-U.S. Gov't]. 2013 Jun;100(7):886–94.

[17] Lo CM, Fan ST, Liu CL, Lai EC, Wong J. Early decision for conversion of laparoscopic to open cholecystectomy for treatment of acute cholecystitis. Am J Surg. 1997 Jun;173(6): 513–7.

[18] Sippey M, Grzybowski M, Manwaring ML, Kasten KR, Chapman WH, Pofahl WE, et al. Acute cholecystitis: risk factors for conversion to an open procedure. J Surg Res. 2015 Dec;199(2):357–61.

[19] Neugebauer E, Troidl H, Kum CK, Eypasch E, Miserez M, Paul A. The E.A.E.S. Consensus Development Conferences on laparoscopic cholecystectomy, appendectomy, and hernia repair. Consensus statements – September 1994. The Educational Committee of the European Association for Endoscopic Surgery. Surg Endosc. [Consensus Development Conference Research Support, Non-U.S. Gov't Review]. 1995 May;9(5):550–63.

[20] Nagle A., J. S. Laparoscopic Cholecystectomy and Choledocholithotomy. In: Blumgart LH, editor. Surgery of the Liver, Biliary Tract, and Pancreas. 4th ed. Philadelphia: Saunders Elsevier; 2007. p. 506–27.

[21] Cannon RM, Brock G, Buell JF. A novel classification system to address financial impact and referral decisions for bile duct injury in laparoscopic cholecystectomy. HPB Surg. 2011;2011:371245.

[22] Vollmer CM, Jr., Callery MP. Biliary injury following laparoscopic cholecystectomy: why still a problem? Gastroenterology. [Comment]. 2007 Sep;133(3):1039–41.

[23] Nijssen MA, Schreinemakers JM, Meyer Z, van der Schelling GP, Crolla RM, Rijken AM. Complications after laparoscopic cholecystectomy: a video evaluation study of whether the critical view of safety was reached. World J Surg. 2015 Jul;39(7):1798–803.

[24] Strasberg SM. Biliary injury in laparoscopic surgery: part 1. Processes used in determination of standard of care in misidentification injuries. Journal of the American College of Surgeons. [Review]. 2005 Oct;201(4):598–603.

[25] Lipman JM, Claridge JA, Haridas M, Martin MD, Yao DC, Grimes KL, et al. Preoperative findings predict conversion from laparoscopic to open cholecystectomy. Surgery. 2007 Oct;142(4):556–63; discussion 63–5.

[26] Pitt SC, Jin LX, Hall BL, Strasberg SM, Pitt HA. Incidental gallbladder cancer at cholecystectomy: when should the surgeon be suspicious? Ann Surg. 2014 Jul;260(1): 128–33.

[27] Schafer M, Krahenbuhl L, Buchler MW. Predictive factors for the type of surgery in acute cholecystitis. Am J Surg. 2001 Sep;182(3):291–7.

[28] Rosen M, Brody F, Ponsky J. Predictive factors for conversion of laparoscopic cholecystectomy. Am J Surg. 2002 Sep;184(3):254–8.

[29] Yang TF, Guo L, Wang Q. Evaluation of preoperative risk factor for converting laparoscopic to open cholecystectomy: a meta-analysis. Hepato-gastroenterology. [Meta-Analysis Review]. 2014 Jun;61(132):958–65.

[30] Licciardello A, Arena M, Nicosia A, Di Stefano B, Cali G, Arena G, et al. Preoperative risk factors for conversion from laparoscopic to open cholecystectomy. Eur Rev Med Pharmacol Sci. 2014 Dec;18(2 Suppl):60–8.

[31] Akcakaya A., Okan I., Bas G., Sahin G., Sachin M. Does the difficulty of laparoscopic cholecystectomy differ between genders? Indian J Surg. 2015;77 (Suppl 2):S452–6.

[32] Donkervoort SC, van Ruler O, Dijksman LM, van Geloven AA, Pierik EG. Identification of risk factors for an unfavorable laparoscopic cholecystectomy course after endoscopic retrograde cholangiography in the treatment of choledocholithiasis. Surg Endosc. 2010 Apr;24(4):798–804.

[33] Simopoulos C, Botaitis S, Karayiannakis AJ, Tripsianis G, Pitiakoudis M, Polychronidis A. The contribution of acute cholecystitis, obesity, and previous abdominal surgery on the outcome of laparoscopic cholecystectomy. Am Surg. 2007 Apr;73(4):371–6.

[34] Yokoe M, Takada T, Strasberg SM, Solomkin JS, Mayumi T, Gomi H, et al. TG13 diagnostic criteria and severity grading of acute cholecystitis (with videos). J Hepatobiliary Pancreat Sci. [Practice Guideline]. 2013 Jan;20(1):35–46.

[35] Cwik G, Skoczylas T, Wyroslak-Najs J, Wallner G. The value of percutaneous ultrasound in predicting conversion from laparoscopic to open cholecystectomy due to acute cholecystitis. Surg Endosc. [Comparative Study]. 2013 Jul;27(7):2561–8.

[36] Paul Wright G, Stilwell K, Johnson J, Hefty MT, Chung MH. Predicting length of stay and conversion to open cholecystectomy for acute cholecystitis using the 2013 Tokyo Guidelines in a US population. J Hepatobiliary Pancreat Sci. 2015 Nov;22(11):795–801.

[37] Asai K, Watanabe M, Kusachi S, Matsukiyo H, Saito T, Kodama H, et al. Risk factors for conversion of laparoscopic cholecystectomy to open surgery associated with the severity characteristics according to the Tokyo guidelines. Surg Today. 2014 Dec;44(12): 2300–4.

[38] Lal P, Agarwal PN, Malik VK, Chakravarti AL. A difficult laparoscopic cholecystectomy that requires conversion to open procedure can be predicted by preoperative ultrasonography. Jsls. 2002 Jan–Mar;6(1):59–63.

[39] Gupta N, Ranjan G, Arora MP, Goswami B, Chaudhary P, Kapur A, et al. Validation of a scoring system to predict difficult laparoscopic cholecystectomy. Int J Surg. 2013;11(9):1002–6.

[40] Stanisic V, Milicevic M, Kocev N, Stojanovic M, Vlaovic D, Babic I, et al. Prediction of difficulties in laparoscopic cholecystectomy on the base of routinely available parameters in a smaller regional hospital. Eur Rev Med Pharmacol Sci. 2014;18(8):1204–11.

[41] Nidoni R, Udachan TV, Sasnur P, Baloorkar R, Sindgikar V, Narasangi B. Predicting difficult laparoscopic cholecystectomy based on clinicoradiological assessment. J Clin Diagn Res. 2015 Dec;9(12):PC09–12.

[42] Bedirli A, Sozuer EM, Yuksel O, Yilmaz Z. Laparoscopic cholecystectomy for symptomatic gallstones in diabetic patients. J Laparoendosc Adv Surg Tech A. 2001 Oct;11(5): 281–4.

[43] Paajanen H, Suuronen S, Nordstrom P, Miettinen P, Niskanen L. Laparoscopic versus open cholecystectomy in diabetic patients and postoperative outcome. Surg Endosc. [Evaluation Studies]. 2011 Mar;25(3):764–70.

[44] Cho JY, Han HS, Yoon YS, Ahn KS. Risk factors for acute cholecystitis and a complicated clinical course in patients with symptomatic cholelithiasis. Arch Surg. 2010 Apr;145(4): 329–33; discussion 33.

[45] Karamanos E, Sivrikoz E, Beale E, Chan L, Inaba K, Demetriades D. Effect of diabetes on outcomes in patients undergoing emergent cholecystectomy for acute cholecystitis. World J Surg. [Evaluation Studies]. 2013 Oct;37(10):2257–64.

[46] Hickman MS, Schwesinger WH, Page CP. Acute cholecystitis in the diabetic. A case-control study of outcome. Arch Surg. [Comparative Study]. 1988 Apr;123(4):409–11.

[47] Walsh DB, Eckhauser FE, Ramsburgh SR, Burney RB. Risk associated with diabetes mellitus in patients undergoing gallbladder surgery. Surgery. 1982 Mar;91(3):254–7.

[48] Shpitz B, Sigal A, Kaufman Z, Dinbar A. Acute cholecystitis in diabetic patients. Am Surg. [Comparative Study]. 1995 Nov;61(11):964–7.

[49] Ibrahim S, Hean TK, Ho LS, Ravintharan T, Chye TN, Chee CH. Risk factors for conversion to open surgery in patients undergoing laparoscopic cholecystectomy. World J Surg. 2006 Sep;30(9):1698–704.

[50] Lee NW, Collins J, Britt R, Britt LD. Evaluation of preoperative risk factors for converting laparoscopic to open cholecystectomy. Am Surg. 2012 Aug;78(8):831–3.

[51] Aziz H, Pandit V, Joseph B, Jie T, Ong E. Age and obesity are independent predictors of bile duct injuries in patients undergoing laparoscopic cholecystectomy. World J Surg. 2015 Jul;39(7):1804–8.

[52] Goonawardena J, Gunnarsson R, de Costa A. Predicting conversion from laparoscopic to open cholecystectomy presented as a probability nomogram based on preoperative patient risk factors. Am J Surg. 2015 Sep;210(3):492–500.

[53] Paajanen H, Kakela P, Suuronen S, Paajanen J, Juvonen P, Pihlajamaki J. Impact of obesity and associated diseases on outcome after laparoscopic cholecystectomy. Surg Laparosc Endosc Percutan Tech. 2012 Dec;22(6):509–13.

[54] Costantini R, Caldaralo F, Palmieri C, Napolitano L, Aceto L, Cellini C, et al. Risk factors for conversion of laparoscopic cholecystectomy. Ann Ital Chir. 2012 May–Jun;83(3):245–52.

[55] Ahn KS, Kim YH, Kang KJ, Kim TS, Cho KB, Kim ES. Impact of preoperative ERCP on laparoscopic cholecystectomy: a case-controlled study with propensity score matching. World J Surg. [Research Support, Non-U.S. Gov't]. 2015 Sep;39(9):2235–42.

[56] Kwon YH, Cho CM, Jung MK, Kim SG, Yoon YK. Risk factors of open converted cholecystectomy for cholelithiasis after endoscopic removal of choledocholithiasis. Dig Dis Sci. 2015 Feb;60(2):550–6.

[57] Beliaev AM, Booth M. Late two-stage laparoscopic cholecystectomy is associated with an increased risk of major bile duct injury. ANZ J Surg. 2016 Jan;86(1–2):63–8.

[58] Boerma D, Rauws EA, Keulemans YC, Janssen IM, Bolwerk CJ, Timmer R, et al. Wait-and-see policy or laparoscopic cholecystectomy after endoscopic sphincterotomy for bile-duct stones: a randomised trial. Lancet. [Clinical Trial Multicenter Study Randomized Controlled Trial Research Support, Non-U.S. Gov't]. 2002 Sep 7;360(9335):761–5.

[59] Maseda E, Maggi G, Gomez-Gil R, Ruiz G, Madero R, Garcia-Perea A, et al. Prevalence of and risk factors for biliary carriage of bacteria showing worrisome and unexpected resistance traits. J Clin Microbiol. 2013 Feb;51(2):518–21.

[60] Reinders JS, Kortram K, Vlaminckx B, van Ramshorst B, Gouma DJ, Boerma D. Incidence of bactobilia increases over time after endoscopic sphincterotomy. Dig Surg. [Multicenter Study Randomized Controlled Trial]. 2011;28(4):288–92.

[61] Hirota M, Takada T, Kawarada Y, Nimura Y, Miura F, Hirata K, et al. Diagnostic criteria and severity assessment of acute cholecystitis: Tokyo Guidelines. J Hepatobiliary Pancreat Surg. [Practice Guideline Research Support, Non-U.S. Gov't]. 2007;14(1):78–82.

[62] Wevers KP, van Westreenen HL, Patijn GA. Laparoscopic cholecystectomy in acute cholecystitis: C-reactive protein level combined with age predicts conversion. Surg Laparosc Endosc Percutan Tech. [Comparative Study]. 2013 Apr;23(2):163–6.

[63] Beliaev AM, Marshall RJ, Booth M. C-reactive protein has a better discriminative power than white cell count in the diagnosis of acute cholecystitis. J Surg Res. 2015 Sep;198(1): 66–72.

[64] Tayeb M, Raza SA, Khan MR, Azami R. Conversion from laparoscopic to open cholecystectomy: multivariate analysis of preoperative risk factors. J Postgrad Med. 2005 Jan–Mar;51(1):17–20; discussion 1–2.

[65] Pejovic T, Stojadinovic MM. Scoring system development and validation for prediction choledocholithiasis before open cholecystectomy. Srp Arh Celok Lek. [Research Support, Non-U.S. Gov't]. 2015 Nov–Dec;143(11–12):681–7.

[66] Kanakala V, Borowski DW, Pellen MG, Dronamraju SS, Woodcock SA, Seymour K, et al. Risk factors in laparoscopic cholecystectomy: a multivariate analysis. Int J Surg. 2011;9(4):318–23.

[67] Yamashita Y, Takada T, Strasberg SM, Pitt HA, Gouma DJ, Garden OJ, et al. TG13 surgical management of acute cholecystitis. J Hepatobiliary Pancreat Sci. [Practice Guideline]. 2013 Jan;20(1):89–96.

[68] Booij KA, de Reuver PR, Nijsse B, Busch OR, van Gulik TM, Gouma DJ. Insufficient safety measures reported in operation notes of complicated laparoscopic cholecystectomies. Surgery. [Evaluation Studies]. 2014 Mar;155(3):384–9.

[69] Strasberg SM, Brunt LM. Rationale and use of the critical view of safety in laparoscopic cholecystectomy. J Am Coll Surg. 2010 Jul;211(1):132–8.

[70] Shingu Y, Komatsu S, Norimizu S, Taguchi Y, Sakamoto E. Laparoscopic subtotal cholecystectomy for severe cholecystitis. Surg Endosc. 2016 Feb;30(2):526–31.

[71] Kaplan D, Inaba K, Chouliaras K, Low GM, Benjamin E, Lam L, et al. Subtotal cholecystectomy and open total cholecystectomy: alternatives in complicated cholecystitis. Am Surg. [Comparative Study Evaluation Studies]. 2014 Oct;80(10):953–5.

[72] Sinha I, Smith ML, Safranek P, Dehn T, Booth M. Laparoscopic subtotal cholecystectomy without cystic duct ligation. Br J Surg. 2007 Dec;94(12):1527–9.

[73] Strasberg SM, Eagon CJ, Drebin JA. The "hidden cystic duct" syndrome and the infundibular technique of laparoscopic cholecystectomy – the danger of the false infundibulum. J Am Coll Surg. 2000 Dec;191(6):661–7.

[74] Strasberg SM. Biliary injury in laparoscopic surgery: part 2. Changing the culture of cholecystectomy. J Am Coll Surg. [Review]. 2005 Oct;201(4):604–11.

[75] Abelson JS, Afaneh C, Rich BS, Dakin G, Zarnegar R, Fahey TJ, 3rd, et al. Advanced laparoscopic fellowship training decreases conversion rates during laparoscopic cholecystectomy for acute biliary diseases: a retrospective cohort study. Int J Surg. 2015 Jan;13:221–6.

[76] Blumgart LH. Stones in the Common Bile Duct – Clinical Features and Open Surgical Approaches and Techniques. In: Blumgart LH, editor. Surgery of the Liver, Biliary Tract, and Pancreas. 4th ed. Philadelphia: Saunders Elsevier; 2007. p. 528–47.

[77] Koc B, Adas G, Karahan S. Use of laparoscopic common bile duct exploration for failed endoscopic bile duct stone extractions. Minerva Chir. 2014 Aug;69(4):209–15.

[78] Alponat A, Kum CK, Koh BC, Rajnakova A, Goh PM. Predictive factors for conversion of laparoscopic cholecystectomy. World J Surg. 1997 Jul–Aug;21(6):629–33.

[79] Afaneh C, Abelson J, Rich BS, Dakin G, Zarnegar R, Barie PS, et al. Obesity does not increase morbidity of laparoscopic cholecystectomy. J Surg Res. 2014 Aug;190(2):491–7.

[80] Andrews S. Does concentration of surgical expertise improve outcomes for laparoscopic cholecystectomy? 9 year audit cycle. Surgeon. 2013 Dec;11(6):309–12.

[81] Giger UF, Michel JM, Opitz I, Th Inderbitzin D, Kocher T, Krahenbuhl L. Risk factors for perioperative complications in patients undergoing laparoscopic cholecystectomy: analysis of 22,953 consecutive cases from the Swiss Association of Laparoscopic and Thoracoscopic Surgery database. J Am Coll Surg. 2006 Nov;203(5):723–8.

[82] Madani A, Watanabe Y, Feldman LS, Vassiliou MC, Barkun JS, Fried GM, et al. Expert intraoperative judgment and decision-making: defining the cognitive competencies for safe laparoscopic cholecystectomy. J Am Coll Surg. [Research Support, Non-U.S. Gov't]. 2015 Nov;221(5):931–40 e8.

[83] Kama NA, Kologlu M, Doganay M, Reis E, Atli M, Dolapci M. A risk score for conversion from laparoscopic to open cholecystectomy. Am J Surg. 2001 Jun;181(6):520–5.

[84] Kologlu M, Tutuncu T, Yuksek YN, Gozalan U, Daglar G, Kama NA. Using a risk score for conversion from laparoscopic to open cholecystectomy in resident training. Surgery. [Validation Studies]. 2004 Mar;135(3):282–7.

[85] Sugrue M, Sahebally SM, Ansaloni L, Zielinski MD. Grading operative findings at laparoscopic cholecystectomy – a new scoring system. World J Emerg Surg. 2015;10:14.

[86] Fry DE, Pine M, Locke D, Pine G. Composite measurement of outcomes in medicare inpatient laparoscopic cholecystectomy. J Am Coll Surg. [Evaluation Studies Research Support, Non-U.S. Gov't]. 2015 Jul;221(1):102–9.

[87] Muller BP, Holzinger F, Leepin H, Klaiber C. Laparoscopic cholecystectomy: quality of care and benchmarking. Results of a single-institution specialized in laparoscopy compared with those of a nationwide study in Switzerland. Surg Endosc. [Comparative Study Validation Studies]. 2003 Feb;17(2):300–5.

[88] Strasberg SM, Hertl M, Soper NJ. An analysis of the problem of biliary injury during laparoscopic cholecystectomy. J Am Coll Surg. [Review]. 1995 Jan;180(1):101–25.

[89] Beliaev AM, Booth M. An association between conversion of laparoscopic cholecystectomy to open surgery and intra-abdominal organ injury. ANZ J Surg. 2016; doi: 10.1111/ans.13539.

[90] Dindo D, Demartines N, Clavien PA. Classification of surgical complications: a new proposal with evaluation in a cohort of 6336 patients and results of a survey. Ann Surg. [Comparative Study Evaluation Studies Validation Studies]. 2004 Aug;240(2):205–13.

[91] Fry DE, Pine M, Pine G. Ninety-day postdischarge outcomes of inpatient elective laparoscopic cholecystectomy. Surgery. [Evaluation Studies]. 2014 Oct;156(4):931–6.

[92] Rana G, Bhullar JS, Subhas G, Kolachalam RB, Mittal VK. Thirty-day readmissions after inpatient laparoscopic cholecystectomy: factors and outcomes. Am J Surg. 2016 Mar; 211(3):626–30.

[93] Harboe KM, Bardram L. The quality of cholecystectomy in Denmark: outcome and risk factors for 20,307 patients from the national database. Surg Endosc. 2011 May;25(5): 1630–41.

Chapter 4

Diagnosis and Management of Rectosigmoid Perforations

Alper Yavuz, Çiğdem Hacifazlioğlu, Gökhan Akkurt,
Altan Aydin and Hakan Ataş

Additional information is available at the end of the chapter

http://dx.doi.org/10.5772/64383

Abstract

Rectosigmoid colon, starting from the descending colon to the anus, having the peritoneal and retroperitoneal parts, is provided through the superior mesenteric artery and the inferior mesenteric artery. Many etiological reasons may be responsible for the perforation of the rectosigmoid colon, which may be usually perforated due to causes of iatrogenic and traumatic origins. The rectosigmoid perforations, which can be diagnosed preoperatively through examination, laboratory, and radiological examinations, may not be detected even in the intraoperative period sometimes. In its treatment, applications, such as conservative approaches, endoclip, laparoscopy, and open surgery, can be performed.

Keywords: rectum, sigmoid colon, perforation

1. Introduction

Rectosigmoid colon perforations are emergency surgery cases that general surgeons may encounter. Some intraperitoneal and retroperitoneal rectosigmoid colon cases develop out of sight away from the pelvis. It may be because of this that serious problems may be experienced in the diagnosis and treatment of the disease. These difficulties cause delayed diagnosis or no diagnosis at all. For this reason, discussing the diagnosis and treatment of rectosigmoid perforation under a separate heading can be important.

2. Sigmoid colon and rectum anatomy

The colon is a part of the gastrointestinal tract ranging between the ileocecal valve and the rectosigmoid junction. It consists of the cecum, ascending colon, transverse colon, descending colon, and the sigmoid colon in that order. The descending colon continues as sigmoid colon at crista iliac level. The sigmoid colon is divided into two sections as 'iliac part', located and constant in the left iliac region, and 'pelvic part', which is mobile. This structure has been named as such because it looks like letter 'S'. Although it varies from person to person, it ends at the third sacral vertebra level. While the iliac part does not have a mesentery, the pelvic part has a mesentery that looks like the Greek letter lambda (Λ λ). The pelvic colon terminates in the rectosigmoid region, and superior rectal veins are located in the sigmoid colon mesentery. While the rectosigmoid compound serves as a functional sphincter, allowing transition of faeces to the rectum by opening up with sigmoid contractions, it prevents stool reflux by closing up during rectal contractions.

The sigmoid colon is the continuation of the descending colon and while its length is variable, it is usually 40 cm. The sigmoid colon, which follows an intraperitoneal course, is in close neighbourhood to the iliac artery and vein, ureter, bladder, uterus, sacral plexus, and the piriformis muscle. The rectum is part of the gastrointestinal system extending between the rectosigmoid junction and the anus and is about 13–15 cm long. The nourishment of the loops of the colon is supplied generally by two main vessels: the superior mesenteric artery (SMA) and the inferior mesenteric artery (IMA) originating from the abdominal aorta. The SMA, which provides nourishment to the small intestine, the cecum, the ascending colon, and the transverse colon, departs from the abdominal aorta right from underneath the celiac trunk, following its course downwards from the rear part of the pancreas and gives out the right colic, middle colic, and ileocolic branches into the colon mesentery. The inferior mesenteric artery (IMA) originating from the infrarenal aorta provides nourishment to the descending colon, the sigmoid colon, and the upper rectum. Major vascular anastomoses are involved in the circulation of the intestines. The vasa recta of the colon are formed by the anastomoses made peripherally between the ileocolic, right, middle, and left colic arteries and the marginal artery of Drummond. The arc of Riolan is described as the anastomosis between the left colic branch of the IMA and the middle colic branches of the SMA. The venous drainage of the colon and rectum is maintained in parallel with the arteries with the exception of the inferior mesenteric vein (IMV). The IMV progresses retroperitoneal behind the pancreas and flows into the splenic vein, allows the venous drainage of the descending colon, the sigmoid colon, and the upper rectum. Autonomic innervation is provided through pre-ganglionic and post-ganglionic sympathetic fibres and lumbar branches of sympathetic chain. The pre-ganglionic parasympathetic fibres are provided through pelvic splanchnic fibre, extending from the S2, S3, and S4 primer ventral ramus. It prevents stool reflux by closing up during contractions [1–3].

Rectum is a part of gastrointestinal system located between rectosigmoid compound and anus and approximately 13–15 cm long. Although there are disagreements between anatomists and surgeons on the identification of the rectosigmoid region, the region where the sigmoid colon turns downwards at the level of promontorium, towards the sacrum concavity, is named as the rectosigmoid corner. Rectum descends down the sacrum concavity 13–15 cm, reaching 2–3 cm below the coccyx. At this level, passing through the levator muscles, it constitutes the anal canal of 3–4 cm long and terminates at the anus. There are also two different identifications of the anal canal: anatomical and surgical. While the anatomical anal canal is the region between the anal verge and the lineadentata, the surgical anal canal is the section of about 3–4 cm between the anal verge and the anorectal ring. Rectum is typically divided into three sections as the upper ⅓, the medium ⅓, and the lower ⅓ of the rectum. In practice, each section is calculated as about 5 cm. The anterior and lateral of the upper ⅓ of the rectum is covered with peritoneum. While the medium ⅓ of the rectum is covered with peritoneum on the anterior, the lower ⅓ of the rectum is below the peritoneal reflection. While the proximal and distal section of the rectum is convex to the right, its middle part is convex to the left. These folds extend towards the lumen as Houston valves, and usually, the middle valve of the Houston is on a line with anterior peritoneal reflection [4, 5]. The rectum descends down forward towards the sacrum concavity from the rectosigmoid junction onward, turns backwards in the direction of the rectum canal from about 2–3 cm below the coccyx, and going through the levator muscles and form the anal canal, ends at the anus. The blood flow to the rectum is maintained by three arteries. While the superior rectal artery that supplies blood flow to the upper and middle section of the rectum is rooted in the IMA, the middle rectal arteries branch out from the internal iliac arteries and the inferior rectal arteries branch out from the internal pudendal arteries. The middle sacral artery originating from the aortal bifurcation is responsible even if only for a little blood supply to the rectum. The venous drainage of the rectum follows the arteries like in the colon but differently from this, they flow into both the portal and the caval system. While the venous drainage of the upper and middle rectum flow into the portal system, that of the lower rectum and the anal canal flow into the caval system [2, 3]. The lymphatic vessels of the upper and middle rectum pour into inferior mesenteric nodes. The lymph flow coming from the lower rectum may also be lateral towards inferior and middle rectal arteries, posterior middle sacral artery, or anterior rectovesical or the canals in rectovaginal septum. While the anal canal lymphatics on the lineadentata pour into the superior rectal lymphatics and the inferior mesenteric lymph nodes, those below the lineadentata pour primarily into inguinal, superior, and inferior rectal lymph nodes. The rectum innervation consists of sympathetic and parasympathetic nerves. The sympathetic nerves taken from the thoracic columnar segment unite under the inferior mesenteric artery and form the inferior mesenteric plexus. The lower rectum, bladder and genital organs take their sympathetic innervation from the hypogastric nerves. The sacral third, fourth, and fifth parasympathetic nerves merge and are named as nervierigentes. Combining with the hypogastric nerves at anterior and lateral of the rectum, they form the pelvic plexus. The internal anal sphincter is innervated by both sympathetic and parasympathetic nerves and the both are inhibitors. The external anal sphincter and the levator muscles are innervated by the inferior rectal branch of the internal pudendal nerve (S2, S3, and S4) and the perineal branch of the fourth sacral nerve [4, 5].

3. Epidemiology

There is not enough data in the literature on the incidence and prevalence of rectum or colon perforations. Studies have been traced especially on perforations occurring as a result of colonoscopic procedures and perforations developing after diverticulitis. While the incidence rate of perforations due to diverticular disease was observed to be around four in 100,000, it is 0.019–0.8% during diagnostic procedures following colonoscopy and 0.10–3% in therapeutic procedures [6, 7].

4. Aetiology and pathogenesis

Because several factors of a varying range are responsible in the aetiology of colon perforations, it is quite difficult to classify. However, colon perforations can be classified as follows according to their aetiologies:

1. Iatrogenic perforations
2. Traumatic perforations
3. Perforations due to malignant or diverticular disease
4. Stercoral perforation
5. Idiopathic perforations
6. Perforations that develop owing to other reasons

While in the past, barium enemas used to play an important role among the iatrogenic causes of colon perforations, today endoscopic and surgical interventions are more commonly observed in the aetiology. While perforation rates were high in diagnostic endoscopic procedures when endoscopic procedures were first put into application, these rates have decreased considerably today, thanks to technological developments and experience. However, with the development and frequent application of therapeutic (stent, excision, and clips) endoscopic procedures, a rise is being observed in perforation rates. When colon perforations following colonoscopy are evaluated according to their locations, they are most frequently observed at the rectosigmoid junction and the sigmoid colon with a rate of 52% followed by the cecum with 17%, ascending colon with 14% descending colon with 8%, transverse colon with 7%, and the rectum with around 1%. Colon injuries during endoscopic procedures usually occur on account of two main reasons. The first of these is mechanical-related injuries and the other is electrocautery-related injuries. Another reason for iatrogenic rectosigmoid injuries is surgical interventions [7–9]. While iatrogenic rectosigmoid perforations are commonly observed following the surgeries of branches such as General Surgery, Gynaecology, and Urology that deal frequently with the abdominal and pelvic regions, iatrogenic colon injuries are rarely observed in the surgeries of branches such as brain surgery and orthopaedics that deal with vertebrae and pelvic bone structures.

Traumatic rectosigmoid injuries develop as a result of direct or indirect traumas depending on how they occur. In indirect traumas, usually the injuring of the rectum by indirect means as a result of blunt or sharp abdominal traumas is observed. In direct traumas, injury occurs through the application of a foreign object or pressure to the rectum and sigmoid colon anally as is particularly seen in homosexuals. Direct traumas can also be observed in the form of the injuring of the colon and rectum by direct means such as receiving a blow to the anal region from a sharp object or firearms or falling on top of sharp objects.

Perforation cases of the rectum and sigmoid colon after malignant diseases or diverticular diseases are frequently observed in the literature. While in malignant diseases, they can be spontaneously perforated as a result of the progression of the tumour and they can also be iatrogenically perforated as a result of endoscopic procedures. Sigmoid colon perforation is observed quite frequently in diverticular diseases. As similar to malignant diseases, perforations in diverticular diseases can also occur spontaneously or iatrogenically as a result of endoscopic procedures [6].

Stercoral perforation, which was first described by Berry in the year 1894, is described as the development of necrosis and perforation on the intestinal wall due to the pressure effect of faecal mass [10]. In stercoral perforations, the area that is ulcerated due to the effect of pressure and the perforated area within this area should be pathologically confirmed. Despite the rare incidence of stercoral perforations, the fact that its distinction from other aetiological causes is not made adequately may lead to wrong diagnoses being made [11].

In the aetiology of rectosigmoid perforations, reasons other than the causes mentioned above, such as systemic lupus erythematosus and Behçet's disease, connective tissue diseases such as rheumatoid arthritis, and infectious conditions like cytomegalovirus do rarely lead to perforations. Among drugs, non-steroid inflammatory drugs and steroids are the drugs that most commonly lead to perforations. Despite such a wide range of aetiological agents being involved in the aetiology of rectosigmoid perforations, sometimes idiopathic perforation cases, the cause of which cannot be determined, are also observed [12–14].

5. Clinical picture

The clinical symptoms of rectosigmoid perforations may involve a wide spectrum. While no clinical symptom is observed in a small perforation with an extra peritoneal localisation, a large perforation with an intraperitoneal localisation can present very severe clinical symptoms. It is quite difficult to make a diagnosis so long as clinical symptoms, such as acute abdomen, rectal bleeding, and tenesmus, which are the clinical triad of colon perforations, are absent. Especially, complaints of pain in the epigastric region and duodenal or gastric ulcer in some cases can make diagnosis even more difficult or can lead to a misdiagnosis [14, 15]. The questioning of aetiological factors is very important in diagnosis. The taking of history, such as a recent colonoscopy, diagnosed diverticular, or malignant colorectal disease or anorectal trauma, can help make a diagnosis. Clinical examination can help in the diagnosis of rectosigmoid perforations. A careful abdominal and rectal examination is very important as a clinical examination. Examination findings such as sensitivity, muscular rigidity, and rebound suggesting acute abdomen in the abdominal examination and rectal blood in the rectal examination or irregular intestinal wall structure suggestive of perforation in the palpation can help in making a diagnosis. Acute abdomen, pneumoperitoneum, or several disease groups that cause rectal complaints should be considered in the differential diagnosis of rectosigmoid perforations and patients should be scrutinised carefully and be examined.

6. Diagnosis

Because rectosigmoid perforations are life-threatening, they require early diagnosis and prompt surgical intervention. Diagnosis can usually be made with clinical findings. However, it may be difficult to clinically detect the location and cause of the perforation due to the symptoms not being specific. Clinical diagnosis can vary depending on conditions such as the size of the perforation, the colonic segment where perforation has taken place, the formation mechanism of the perforation, peritoneal contamination, and the underlying colonic pathology. Just as it can be asymptomatic, symptoms and findings can present at the moment of perforation or late. Generally speaking, perforation findings include general or localised abdominal pain, nausea/vomiting, fever, shortness of breath, and chest pain [16, 17].

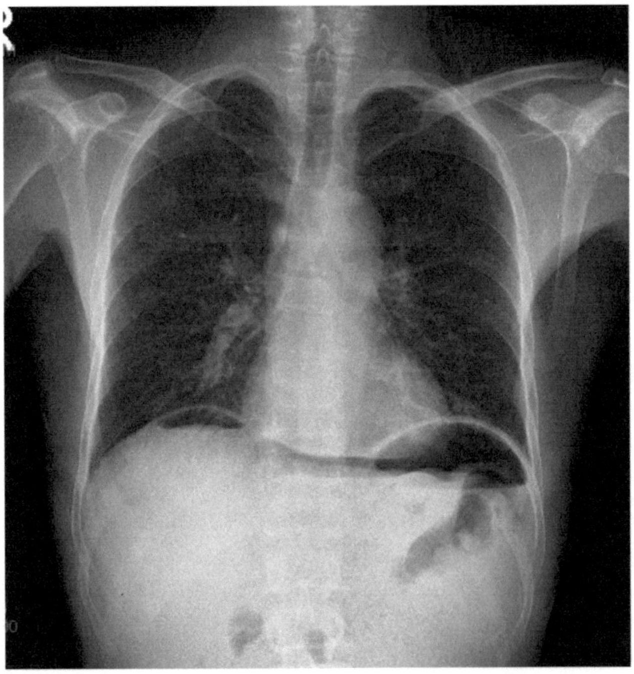

Figure 1. Chest X-Ray showing collection of air in the right subdiaphragmatic space.

The basic question in imaging is revealing the location and the cause of perforation. The first choice in modality of imaging in patients with suspected perforation is direct radiography. In conventional radiography, observing free air inside the peritoneum indicates perforation, but the location and the cause of the perforation cannot be determined (**Figure 1**). Also, small amounts of air may not be detected in radiographies. For the findings of direct radiography to be normal does not exclude the possibility of perforation [16–19]. In the case of suspected perforation, an abdominal graphy and lung graphy are done standing or in the left lateral decubitus position. In the case of perforation, the free air outside the colon can move into the retroperitoneal region and cause subcutaneous emphysema in the scrotum, chest, axilla, and neck. In direct graphies, air beneath the diaphragm, retroperitoneal air, pneumomediastinum, pneumothorax, and subcutaneous air is investigated. Lateral graphies are more sensitive in detecting free air than PA graphies. In left lateral decubitus graphy, air between the liver and the abdominal wall can easily be discerned. In lateral chest graphy, air beneath the diaphragm can be clearly observed. In direct graphies, air inside the subhepatic and perihepatic spaces in the upper quadrant, in the Morrison pouch can be detected. The double wall appearance known as the Rigler sign, air under the central part of the diaphragm known as the Cupola sign and a large amount of air inside the peritoneal cavity known as the Football sign can be detected in direct radiographies [17, 18].

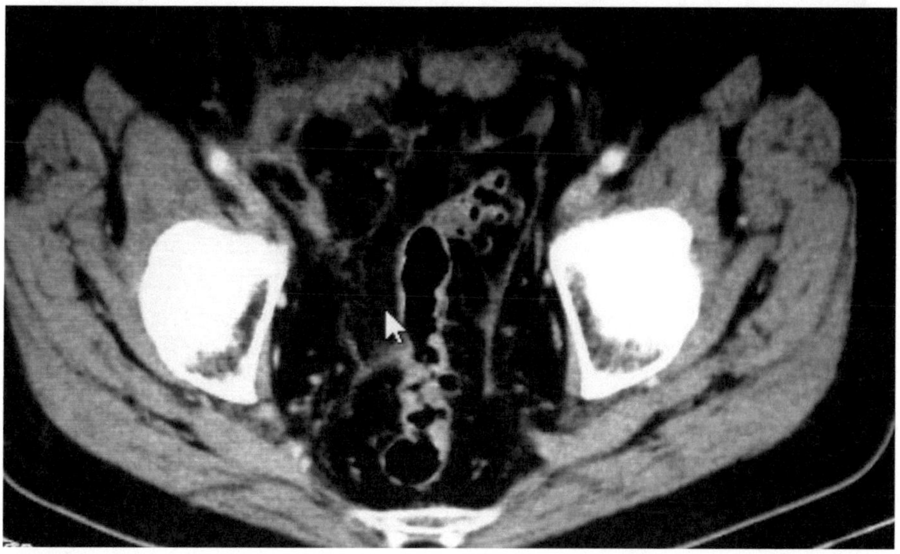

Figure 2. Abdominal CT showing sigmoid diverticular disease and indirect signs of perforation (mesenteric contamination and heterogeneity).

The other method used in the diagnosis of perforation is ultrasonography. It provides fast and easy scanning. It does not include radiation and, therefore, can be preferred in children and in pregnant women. It can detect intraabdominal free or loculated fluid. Also, ultrasonography provides additional diagnostic information. There are studies which state that pneumoperitoneum can be detected with ultrasonography. However, there are also studies stating that it is inadequate due to abdominal gas. For this reason, it has a low diagnostic value when compared with CT [19, 20].

Direct graphies and ultrasonography, when compared with CT, are suboptimal in the evaluation of perforation. CT has been accepted as the best imaging method in revealing the presence, location, cause, and complications (such as phlegmon, abscesses, and peritonitis) of a perforation. Oral and IV contrast agents can be used. The entire abdomen from the pelvis to the upper section of the diaphragm can be scanned with thin slice thickness. The three-dimensional (3D) images can be obtained through multiplanar reconstructions. In the diagnosis of perforation, there are direct and indirect findings of CT (**Figures 2** and **3**). Extraluminal air and contrast agent and intestinal wall discontinuation are direct findings, whereas a phlegmon, abscess, or inflammatory mass related or unrelated to the intestinal wall are indirect findings [20, 21]

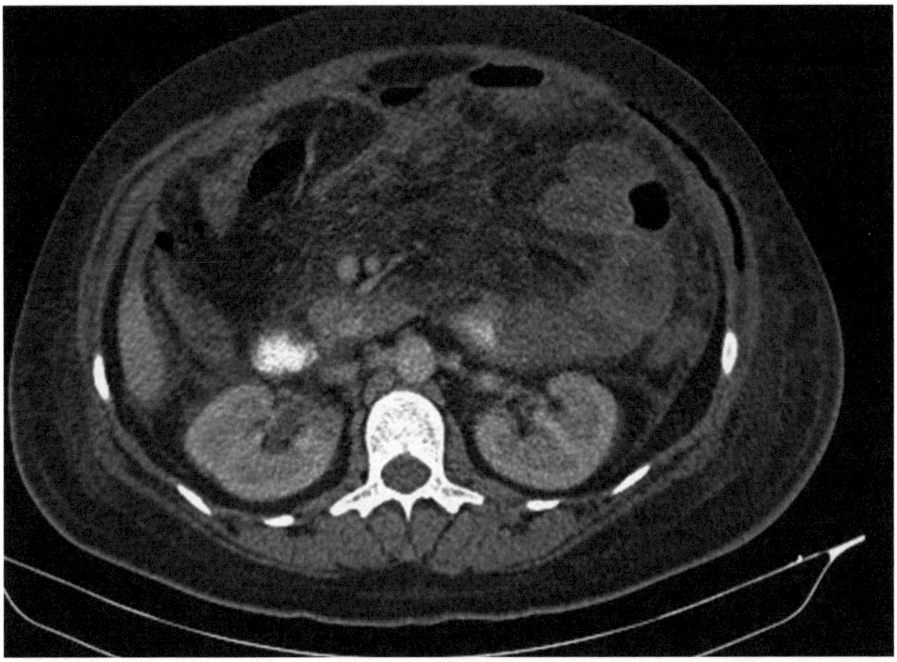

Figure 3. Abdominal CT showing the air in abdominal muscle because of close perforation of sigmoid colon.

The diagnosis of rectosigmoid perforations sometimes can be very difficult in the pre-operative period. In fact, sometimes perforations cannot be observed even intraoperatively. In case of presence of findings suggesting intestinal perforation (gas in the stomach and intestinal content) if perforation focuses cannot be observed, rectosigmoid perforations should be definitely investigated. In the first place, any perforation should be tried to be detected visually, and if no perforation is detected, the pelvic region should be filled with saline and gas bubbles that may come out through manipulation of rectosigmoid should be examined. If no perforation focuses are observed, it is not an indication of absence of perforation. For hidden and small perforation focus, the rectum should be filled with methylene blue (about 250 cc) and possible leakage area should be investigated again by manipulating the rectosigmoid (**Figure 4**).

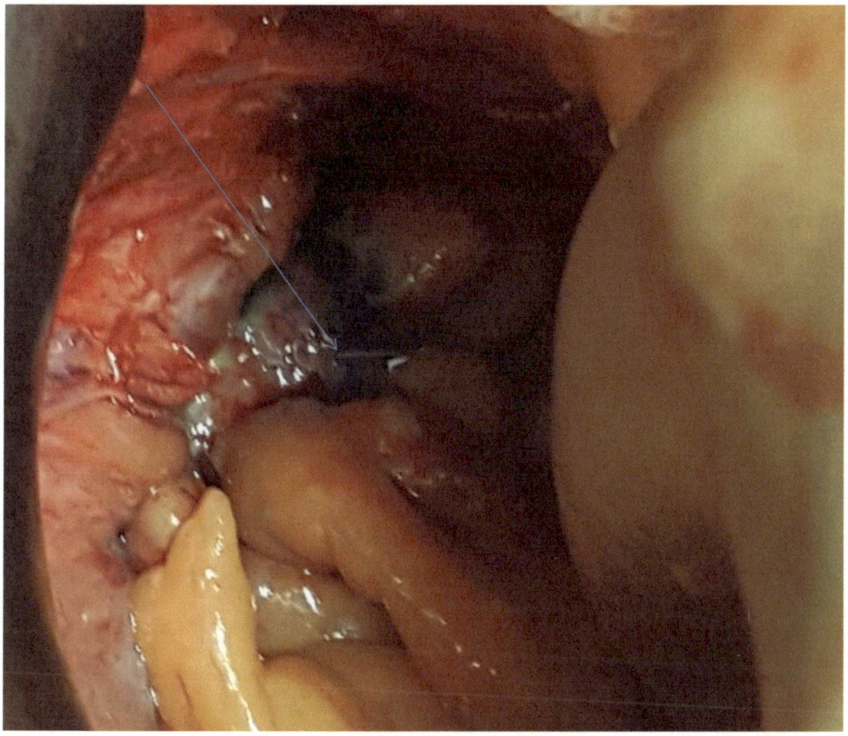

Figure 4. Microperforation only be demonstrated by the way given transanal methylene blue.

7. Treatment

A wide range of treatment options is available from a conservative treatment option to a wide intestinal resection and stoma in the treatment of rectosigmoid perforations. However, the real debate is what treatment will be applied to whom. The way the perforation occurred, its location, diameter, the condition of the intestines, the amount of time that passed after the perforation, the underlying disease, the level of intraabdominal contamination, and the clinical laboratory and radiological findings of the patient gives the physician insight on which treatment option will be applied.

The conservative treatment option is included among colon perforation treatment options due to it shortening the length of hospital stay and decreasing mortality rates. However, for conservative treatment, there must first be an appropriate patient selection and an intensive care unit that can provide adequate support in the unit where it will be applied and a radiological unit must be present. Because these patients must be able to be monitored and given radiological examinations at any hour of the day when necessary [9, 22].

The form of treatment that is usually recommended for rectosigmoid perforations is immediate surgical intervention. The findings detected during the surgery provide guidance on the type of surgery. The form of surgery applied is usually the repairment of the perforation and resection of the perforated area. It is decided according to the level of contamination and the condition of the tissues whether a stoma will be done or not. In the case of more than 24 h having passed after the perforation and a perforation size of more than 2 cm, usually faecal diversion surgeries are recommended [23].

Just as with technological development is used in the treatment of several diseases, laparoscopy is also widely used in the treatment of rectosigmoid perforations. Several surgical techniques such as primary repair resection and faecal diversion which are performed in open surgeries can also be performed laparoscopically. Early return to work and reduced infection and pain are important advantages provided to patients by laparoscopy.

Another minimally invasive technique used in the treatment of rectosigmoid perforations is the repair of perforations with endoscopic approaches. The most commonly used method in this form of treatment is repair of the perforation with an endoscopic clip. In this form of treatment, the size of the perforation, and the experience of the endoscopist performing it are very important [24].

8. Conclusion

Rectosigmoid perforations are seen rarely. The most frequent causes in the aetiology are malignant or diverticular diseases and iatrogenic and traumatic perforations. Clinical examination is very important, but sometimes, diagnosis can be very difficult in spite of advanced assays. Non-invasive or minimal invasive procedures should be the first choice for the treatment, but the selection of a suitable case, of course, is very important.

Author details

Alper Yavuz[1*], Çiğdem Hacifazlioğlu[2], Gökhan Akkurt[1], Altan Aydin[1] and Hakan Ataş[1]

*Address all correspondence to: alperyavuz@hotmail.com

1 General Surgery Department, Kecioren Research and Training Hospital, Ankara, Turkey

2 Radiology Department, Kecioren Research and Training Hospital, Ankara, Turkey

References

[1] Shafik A. Sigmoido-rectal junction reflex. Role in the defecation mechanism. Clin Anat 9:391–394, 1996.

[2] Dunn KMB, Rothenberger DA. Chapter 29. Colon, Rectum, Anus. In: Brunicardi F, Andersen DK, Billiar TR, Dunn DL, Hunter JG, Matthews JB, Pollock RE. eds. Schwartz's Principles of Surgery, 10e. New York, NY: McGraw-Hill; 2015.

[3] Corman ML, Allison SI, Kuehne PJ. Chapter 1. Anatomy and Embryology of the Anus, Rectum and Colon. Colon & Rectal Surgery, Fourth Edition. (Ö. Alabaz, Aygen E, trans). Adana: Nobel Tıp Kitapevi; 2004.

[4] Kodner IJ, Robert D. Colon, Rectum and Anus, Principles of Surgery, Schwartz. 1284 90, 1999.

[5] Romolo J.L. Embryology and anatomy of the colon. Shackelford's Surgery of the Alimentary Tract, 4: 3–16, Philadelphia, 1996.

[6] Morris CR, Harvey IM, Stebbings WS, Speakman CT, Kennedy HJ, Hart AR. Epidemiology of perforated colonic diverticular disease. Postgrad Med J. 2002;78:654–658.

[7] Lohsiriwat V. Colonoscopic perforation: incidence, risk factors, management and outcome. World J Gastroenterol. 2010; 28:16:425–430.

[8] Tam MS, Abbas MA. Perforation following colorectal endoscopy: what happens beyond the endoscopy suite?. Perm J 2013;17:17–21.

[9] Cai SL, Chen T, Yao LQ, Zhong YS. Management of iatrogenic colorectal perforation: From surgery to endoscopy. World J Gastrointest Endosc. 2015;7:819–823.

[10] Berry J. Dilatation and rupture of the sigmoid flexure. Br Med J. 1894;1:301.

[11] Maurer CA, Renzulli P, Mazzucchelli L, Egger B, Seiler CA, Buchler MW. Use of accurate diagnostic criteria may increase incidence of stercoral perforation of the colon. Dis Colon Rectum 2000;43:991– 998.

[12] Yaman İ, Kara C, Karabuğa T, Sözütek A, Tansuğ T, Bozdağ AD, Nazlı O. Nontravmatikkolonperforasyonluhastalarınklinikdeğerlendirilmesivetedavisonuçları. Kolon Rektum Hast Derg 2010; 20:11–18.

[13] Tachikawa Y, Nozawa H, Tanaka J, Nishikawa T, Tanaka T, Kiyomatsu T, Hata K, Kawai K, Kazama S, Yamaguchi H, Ishihara S, Sunami E, Kitayama J, Fujisawa M, Takahashi K, Sakaguchi Y, Ushiku T, Fukayama M, Watanabe T. Colonic perforation in a patient with systemic lupus erythematosus accompanied by cytomegalovirus infection: A case report. Int J Surg Case Rep. 2016;23:70–73.

[14] Yavuz A, Şeker D, Buluş H, Aydın A. Recto-sigmoid perforation mimicking peptic ulcer perforation: a case report. Turkish J Surg. 2011; 27:243–245.

[15] Olnick HM, Harris CM. Spontaneous perforation of the colon. South Med J. 1980;73(3): 326–328.

[16] Cho KC, Baker SR. Extraluminal air. Diagnosis and significance. Radiol Clin North Am 1994;32:829–844.

[17] Rice RP, Thompson WM, Gedgaudas RK. The diagnosis and significance of extraluminal gas in the abdomen. Radiol Clin North Am 1982;20:819–837.

[18] Ghahremani GG. Radiologic evaluation of suspected gastrointestinal perforations. Radiol Clin North Am 1993;31:1219–1234

[19] Stapakis JC, Thickman D (1992) Diagnosis of pneumoperitoneum: abdominal CT vs. upright chest film. J Comput Assist Tomogr 16:713–716

[20] Maniatis V, Chryssikopoulos H, Roussakis A, et al. (2000) Perforation of the alimentary tract: evaluation with computed tomography. Abdom Imaging 25:373–379.

[21] Miki T, Ogata S, Uto M, et al. (2004) Multidetector-row CT findings of colonic perforation: direct visualization of ruptured colonic wall. Abdom Imaging 29:659–662.

[22] Iqbal CW, Chun YS, Farley DR. Colonoscopic perforations: a retrospective review. J Gastrointest Surg 2005; 9: 1229–1235.

[23] Rotholtz NA, Laporte M, Lencinas S, Bun M, Canelas A, Mezzadri N. Laparoscopic approach to colonic perforation due to colonoscopy. World J Surg. 2010;34:1949–1953.

[24] Kim JS, Kim BW, Kim JI, Kim JH, Kim SW, Ji JS, Lee BI, Choi H. Endoscopic clip closure versus surgery for the treatment of iatrogenic colon perforations developed during diagnostic colonoscopy: a review of 115,285 patients. Surg Endosc. 2013;27:501–504.

Chapter 5

Gastrointestinal Foreign Bodies

Obinna Obinwa, David Cooper,
James M. O'Riordan and Paul Neary

Additional information is available at the end of the chapter

http://dx.doi.org/10.5772/63464

Abstract

Retained foreign bodies within the gastrointestinal tract (GIT) are common emergency presentations. The majority will pass spontaneously or be removed endoscopically, but a few selected cases may require emergency surgery for removal. This chapter reviews the management of foreign bodies within the GIT including both instances of foreign body ingestions and foreign body insertions. The scope of this chapter is not limited to evidence-based data on selection of cases for conservative management but also includes data on endoscopic and surgical management.

Keywords: complications, decision support techniques, diagnosis, emergency management, endoscopy, foreign bodies, gastrointestinal tract, humans, surgery

1. Introduction

Gastrointestinal tract (GIT) foreign body ingestions or insertions are common clinical scenarios, with an estimated 1500–2750 patients dying annually from ingested foreign bodies in the United States each year [1–3]. The problem is encountered in all age groups, and the choice of an appropriate technique for removal may, at times, pose a dilemma for the clinician. Although recent reports suggest that most cases of foreign body ingestion do not result in mortality or significant clinical sequelae [4], evidence-based criteria for management should be employed so as to reduce the risk of potential adverse events. Importantly, cases selected for surgical removal should be appropriately investigated and managed.

2. Epidemiology

Foreign body ingestion is more prevalent amongst the paediatric age group than in the adult population. The peak incidence is between 6 months and 6 years [4]. The ingestion of foreign bodies is rarely seen in adults; is accidental and is commonly observed in the form of food (meat and bone) ingestion [5]. High-risk groups among an adult patient population include those with psychiatric disorders, prisoners and intoxicated patients [4]. Intentionally ingested objects typically include common household items (e.g., pens, plastic spoons, toothbrushes or pencils), whereas accidentally ingested items are often food impactions or bones.

Foreign body insertion, on the other hand, especially involving the lower GIT, is more prevalent in an adult demographic [6]. The true incidence is not known, as many patients do not seek medical attention or management is underreported for obvious reasons [7]. These cases are not limited to a particular demographic, and rectal foreign bodies have been reported in patients of all ages, genders and ethnicities [5, 8]. The mean age at presentation is 44 years but ranges from 20 to over 90 years, with a decidedly higher proportion of male patients (17–37:1) [7]. The most common reason for insertion is anal eroticism, with other reasons, in decreasing order of frequency, being concealment (as in prisoners), attention-seeking behaviour, assault and "therapeutic" (i.e., attempts to alleviate constipation) [9]. Some literature reports a bimodal age distribution, with the second peak occurring in males in their sixties, often for breaking up faecal impactions or prostatic massage [10].

3. Surgical pathophysiology

A rational approach to management of gastrointestinal intestinal foreign bodies requires an understanding of the natural course of these ingested or inserted objects. This knowledge is essential to be able to define groups of patients who would require early intervention. Approximately 63–76% of intentionally ingested foreign bodies are removed endoscopically, and the need for surgical intervention ranges from 12 to 16% [4].

Historically, 80% or more of ingested foreign bodies pass spontaneously without the need for intervention [11]. Complications such as impaction, perforation or obstruction occur at areas of physiological narrowing or angulations [12]. Areas of narrowing in the GIT include the upper oesophageal sphincter, aortic arch, left main stem bronchus, lower oesophageal sphincter, pylorus, ileocecal valve and anus; the duodenal sweep is an example of GI angulation [12]. Once foreign bodies have passed through the oesophagus, which is the least expansile aspect of the GIT, most objects pass within 4–6 days or in rare cases in up to 4 weeks [12]. Any anatomical variation in the GIT can alter these series of physiological narrowing and angulations. Therefore, patients with congenital malformations or those who have undergone previous GI surgery are more susceptible to retained foreign bodies [4].

http://dx.doi.org/10.5772/63464

The risk of retention and subsequent complications also varies according to the nature of the foreign body. For example, sharp or pointed objects, fish/animal bones, foil from blister packs, as well as magnets, are associated with an increased risk of perforation [4]. Magnets are especially dangerous as they may attract other simultaneously ingested foreign bodies [13]. Due to their magnetic forces, the objects may adhere to one another across two separate parts of the GI tract leading to severe and potentially fatal complications including volvulus and obstruction, pressure necrosis, fistula formation and perforation [14].

Impaction and progressive erosion of the foreign body through the intestinal wall lead to perforation, and, in most cases, this site of perforation is covered by fibrin, omentum or adjacent loops of bowel [12]. The passage of large amounts of intraluminal air into the peritoneal cavity rarely occurs as a result [12]. Retained gastric, intestinal and rectal foreign objects can cause severe injury through this mechanism. The main site of obstruction for rectal foreign bodies is the mid-rectum as objects are unable to renegotiate the anterior angulation of the rectum. All such retained foreign bodies should, therefore, be treated as potentially hazardous [8].

4. Classifications

A clinical classification of gastrointestinal foreign objects into oesophageal, gastric, intestinal or colorectal foreign bodies is based on the location of the object within the GIT. Objects may also be classified as ingested foreign objects or foreign body insertions using the mechanism of entry as criteria for classification. Further sub-classifications of ingested foreign objects into groups of blunt objects, sharp pointed objects, long objects, food bolus impaction and objects containing poisons are useful in defining the management approach [12].

Foreign body insertions into the rectum may be voluntary or involuntary. The intent may be sexual or non-sexual. Using this two-tier classification system, rectal foreign bodies are classified as voluntary sexual, voluntary non-sexual, involuntary sexual and involuntary non-sexual. The most common category of inserted objects is that of voluntary sexual insertions and includes plastic/glass bottles, vegetables, wooden or rubber objects and sex toys [15]. Cases of insertion of involuntary sexual foreign bodies are almost exclusively limited to the domain of rape and sexual assault [15]. Involuntary non-sexual insertions (e.g., thermometers and enema tips) are found in the elderly, children or the mentally ill, and are often accidental [15]. The term "body packing" represents a form of voluntary non-sexual insertion and refers to smuggling of drugs by concealment in the GIT [12]. For example, illegal drugs (most often cocaine or heroin) are packed within latex condoms or balloons and are swallowed or inserted into the rectum in several parcels [12, 16]. These parcels pose a significant health risk as intoxication secondary to rupture can be potentially fatal. Alternatively, the American Association for the Surgery of Trauma Rectum Injury Scale may be used to assess injury from rectal foreign bodies [7].

5. Clinical presentations and assessment

Patients with gastrointestinal foreign bodies (either inserted or ingested) are often asymptomatic. Alternatively, they may present with a broad range of symptoms, which, vary based on the location, physical characteristics and the content of the object [5]. Most rectal foreign objects are introduced through the anus; however, sometimes, a foreign body is swallowed, fails to pass fully through the GIT, and is held up in the mid-rectum [10]. Patients with foreign bodies introduced through the anus are often embarrassed about their condition and may be reluctant to seek medical care [17]. In most cases, the patients present to the emergency room after failed efforts to remove the object at home [8]. The time interval from insertion to hospital presentation varies, and may be up to 2 weeks [9].

The medical history is highly critical in the management of foreign body ingestion or insertion [5]. The planning of diagnostic workup and the extent and urgency of a possible intervention are primarily decided according to the information provided by the patient regarding the type of object inserted, together with clinical complaints and findings [5]. However, the main difficulty encountered is that of patients' reluctance to divulge the nature of insertion/ingestion. For example, patients with rectal foreign bodies are often embarrassed about their condition and may seek to conceal some relevant facts leading to extensive workups and further delays [18]. A high index of suspicion is required to accurately diagnose their condition. At the same time, the practitioner should try to establish the mechanism of insertion. In one case report, the rectal injury was caused not by the foreign object itself, but by another object used as an introducer [19].

It is pivotal to maintain professionalism and courtesy while simultaneously obtaining an accurate, detailed history. For communicative adults, history of ingestion including timing, type of ingested foreign body and onset of symptoms are often reliable [20]. One must also consider whether such case of involuntary insertion constitutes an assault, for the management of the latter requires other medicolegal considerations. For example, it is essential to keep medical photographs of retrieved rectal foreign bodies for clinical records in cases of assault and child abuse [6]. The clinician should also be prepared to provide emotional support for the patient, and have a chaperone in the room when performing the physical examination [7].

Even in good historians, physical examination is mandatory to out rule potentially hazardous complications such as small-bowel obstruction or perforation. Signs of GI perforation may include tachycardia, subcutaneous crepitus and peritonitis. A medical consultation is required if systemic toxicity is due to ingestion of foreign objects [4]. A respiratory examination is necessary to assess for the presence of wheezing or crepitations suggestive of tracheal compression or aspiration, respectively. Specific other presentations are based on the anatomical region where the foreign body is located.

5.1. Oesophageal foreign bodies

Patients with oesophageal foreign bodies, particularly impacted food boluses, can specify the onset of symptoms and if symptomatic may attempt to localise their discomfort exactly.

However, the area of discomfort does not always accurately correlate with the site of impaction [4]. The typical complaints in symptomatic patients include a vague report of the sensation of something stuck in the centre of the chest or sudden onset of the difficulty of swallowing during eating. If they report the same sensation in the epigastric region, it may indicate that the foreign body has passed the lower oesophageal sphincter. When the foreign body has passed the oesophagus, the majority of patients remain asymptomatic but a sensation of foreign body, with dysphagia, can persist for several hours and thus can mimic a persisting foreign body impaction [12].

Dysphagia is another commonly reported symptom, and in the presence of drooling, especially in paediatric cases, may indicate an oesophageal obstruction. Patients with oesophageal foreign bodies may also present with respiratory symptoms such as a cough, stridor or dyspnea. These symptoms may occur as a result of a direct tracheal compression by the foreign body or indirectly due to aspiration of secretions. Non-specific symptoms, such as abdominal pain or distension, nausea and vomiting, haematemesis or melaena, may be present. If the pericardium and myocardium are involved, the patient may present with acute onset chest pain secondary to mediastinitis or may complain of dyspnoea or severe odynophagia. Such cases are associated with significant morbidity and are recognized causes of mortality [21].

5.2. Gastric and intestinal foreign bodies

Once foreign bodies have passed through the oesophagus, they are usually asymptomatic, unless obstruction or perforation occurs. Symptoms suggestive of obstruction include abdominal pain, distension, vomiting and constipation. The presence of severe abdominal pain that is intensified by movement, fever and/or rigors makes a diagnosis of gastric or small-bowel perforation more likely. The clinician may also be able to predict the level of obstruction based on clinical history alone. For example, in small-bowel obstruction, the pain tends to be colicky in nature, as opposed to large-bowel obstruction that is usually associated with a more constant pain. For more proximal obstructions, vomiting tends to present before constipation, whereas the opposite is more consistent with distal GIT obstructions. Non-bilious vomiting indicates that the obstruction is above the level of the ampulla of Vater. Bilious vomiting occurs when the blockage is below this level, and faecal vomiting is more indicative of distal bowel obstruction. In the presence of obstruction or perforation, the typical findings on physical examination include abdominal distension and tenderness; additional peritoneal signs of rigidity or rebound tenderness make the diagnosis of perforation more likely.

5.3. Colorectal foreign bodies

Because of the wide variety of objects and the variation in trauma caused to local tissues of the rectum and distal colon, a systematic approach to the diagnosis and management of rectal foreign bodies is essential [15]. Common complaints include rectal or abdominal pain, constipation or obstipation, bright red blood per rectum or incontinence. Complications such as bowel obstruction may also occur [6]. Sudden, excruciating pain during defecation should arouse suspicion of a penetrating foreign body that is usually lodged at or just above the anorectal junction [7]. The presence of a chocolate malodorous rectal mucoid discharge signifies necrosis, perforation and/or sepsis [6]. Other manifestations depend on the size and shape of the foreign body, its duration in situ and the presence of infection or perforation.

Physical examination should include a careful abdominal examination to assess for signs of peritonitis or the ability to palpate an object trans-abdominally [15]. Abdominal examination is usually followed by a digital rectal examination. However, some authors advise that an abdominal X-ray should be performed before the rectal examination to prevent inadvertent, accidental injury to the surgeon from sharp objects [15]. A digital rectal examination estimates the distance of the foreign body from the anal verge, as well as assesses sphincter integrity. Sphincter injury is rare in cases of voluntary insertion. However, muscular spasm induced by the foreign body may result in increased sphincter tone. The sphincter may have obvious damage with visible injury to both the internal and external components and should be carefully examined [15]. Most foreign bodies are usually palpable on the digital rectal examination as they are most commonly lodged in the mid rectum.

6. Further investigations/workup

Radiological assessment is the key to further evaluation following a thorough history and clinical examination. For anorectal foreign bodies above the sacral curve and rectosigmoid junction, further evaluation with rigid or flexible proctosigmoidoscopy should be performed if the rectal object is not palpable. Laboratory tests are of limited value and should be limited to a basic pre-operative work, allowing for timely surgical management if appropriate [7, 15]. Patients with peritonitis or perforation should be kept nil by mouth and resuscitated with intravenous fluids and antibiotics [15]. A nasogastric tube should be considered, and Foley's catheter should also be passed [15]. Anti-thromboembolic prophylaxis should be commenced early and continued until discharge, particularly in elderly patients.

Plain radiographs are the first line radiological investigation as they are inexpensive and associated with reduced radiation exposure. Most true foreign bodies are radio-opaque but smaller thinner objects are not always detected [12]. Metal objects tend to be easily identified, whereas small bone or glass or wooden objects are less readily detected. Serial radiographic studies can be used to determine the passage of the foreign body and the complications resulting from it [5]. Biplanar imaging may be necessary if the history suggests foreign body ingestion but there is nothing detected on initial plain radiograph [12]. Complications such as aspiration, free mediastinal/peritoneal air or subcutaneous emphysema may also be detected on chest X-ray in a limited number of cases [12]. X-ray is not sufficient and not required in patients with non-bony food bolus impaction and without clinical signs of perforation [12].

The use of barium swallow as part of the workup for a patient with ingested foreign body is not advised [12]. It is associated with an increased risk of aspiration and may obscure visualization if subsequent endoscopy is indicated. If an upper GI foreign body is not detected on plain films, then an oral contrast medium (e.g., gastrograffin) may be considered, assuming oesophageal obstruction has been out ruled [12]. Computed tomography (CT) of the abdomen and pelvis is especially useful when radiolucent materials cannot be detected with plain X-rays [5]. It may also be considered if the rectal foreign body has been in place for more than 24 h [8]. This modality has largely supplanted the previous contrast studies. The risk of potential complications increases if the foreign body has been in place for more than 24 h. With CT, the shape, size, location and depth of the impacted foreign body and the surrounding tissue can be visualized, which is important in determining treatment. Of note, free intraperitoneal air is a poor radiological sign [12]. The region of perforation can be identified on CT scan as a thickened intestinal segment, localized pneumoperitoneum, regional fatty infiltration or associated obstruction [12, 22].

7. Further management

7.1. Ingested foreign objects

Conservative outpatient management, on the one hand, is appropriate for asymptomatic patients with blunt objects in the stomach that are smaller than 2–2.5 cm in diameter and 5–6 cm in length [12]. As a rule, objects greater than 2.5 cm in diameter will rarely pass through the pylorus or ileocecal valve and objects longer than 6 cm will also rarely pass through the duodenal sweep [12]. Patients who are to be managed conservatively should be educated about the symptoms of potential complications and instructed to represent if they occur [12]. Of particular importance are those related to perforation or obstruction. They should also be instructed to check their bowel motions to monitor for spontaneous passage of the foreign body [12]. If the foreign body fails to pass beyond the stomach within 4 weeks, it is likely to require intervention [4, 12]. Conservative in-patient management, on the other hand, is recommended for "body-packers" with a failure rate of only 2–5% [12]. The management comprises clinical observation, whole bowel irrigation and radiographic follow-up for observing passage of the parcels [12].

Recently, the European Society of Gastrointestinal Endoscopy (ESGE) published guidelines for foreign body management [12]. According to their guidelines, the timing of endoscopic intervention is divided into three groups: emergency, urgent and non-urgent. Patients who are unable to manage their secretions on presentation, those who swallowed disk batteries and those with sharp objects in the oesophagus will require emergent endoscopic intervention (preferably within 2 h, but at latest within 6 h) [12]. Urgent (within 24 h) endoscopy is recommended for removal of oesophageal foreign objects that are not sharp-pointed, food impaction without complete obstruction, sharp pointed objects in the stomach or duodenum and objects longer than 6 cm in length and magnets within endoscopic reach [12]. As delay decreases the likelihood of successful removal of such objects and increases the risk of complication, endoscopic removal should not be delayed beyond 72 h even for the non-urgent cases [12]. Cases suitable for non-urgent management include coins in the oesophagus which may be observed for 12–24 h before endoscopic removal in an asymptomatic patient [4]. Cylindrical and disk batteries that are in the stomach of patients without signs of GI injury may be observed for as long as 48 h before proceeding with endoscopic removal [4]. Batteries remaining in the stomach longer than 48 h should be removed before 72 h as well as objects in the stomach with a diameter greater than 2.5 cm [4].

In practice, conscious sedation may be used for endoscopic removal in adults, but endotracheal intubation under general anaesthesia is often required for objects that are harder to remove. Standard-sized overtubes that extend past the upper oesophageal sphincter not only protect the airways but also facilitate passage of the endoscope during removal of multiple sharp, pointed objects or piecemeal extraction of an impacted food bolus [12]. Overtubes help to reduce further potential damage to the mucosa of the GIT while the foreign body is being withdrawn. The specific example of removal of food bolus may simply involve gently pushing the bolus into the stomach with success rates of over 90% and minimal complications [12]. However, extraction may also be performed using grasping forceps, retrieval graspers, polypectomy snare, basket and retrieval nets. Other blunt objects such as coins, buttons, toys, batteries and magnets can also be removed using a similar range of retrieval devices. Long objects including strings, cords, pen, pencils, toothbrushes, cutlery and screwdrivers are best removed using polypectomy snares or baskets. A transparent cap and latex rubber hood may be required additionally for removal of sharp pointed objects. If the foreign body cannot safely be retrieved endoscopically, in-patient treatment and close clinical observation are mandatory.

Bleeding can also be encountered as a complication of ingestion or endoscopic removal of sharp pointed objects. The principle of successful management is by meticulous resuscitation, accurate endoscopic diagnosis and timely application of appropriate therapy. The endoscopic and surgical management is similar to that of bleeding peptic ulcers. For example, ulcers with a clean base or non-protuberant pigmented dot in an ulcer bed, which are at low risk of re-bleeding, do not require endoscopic treatment [23]. For all others, including those who have active bleeding or non-bleeding visible vessels or have adherent blood clot, endoscopic treatment should be administered [23]. Injection with 1:10,000 adrenaline around the bleeding point and then into the bleeding vessel achieves haemostasis in up to 95% of cases [23]. Additional injection of sclerosants or absolute alcohol does not confer additional benefit. Fibrin glue and thrombin may be more effective, but they are not widely available. Heater probes, multipolar coagulation (BICAP), argon plasma coagulation or mechanical clips may also be used but consulting a gastroenterologist may be more appropriate at this stage. Repeat therapeutic endoscopy may be attempted if there is a suggestion of further active bleeding or in cases where the initial endoscopic treatment was sub-optimal. Operative intervention is mandatory if initial control of bleeding is not possible endoscopically and techniques are as described in standard surgical texts.

Besides for failure to control bleeding endoscopically, there are other indications for surgical intervention. Urgent cases include cases of ruptured narcotic packets or leakage, presentations with clinical evidence of peritonitis and intestinal obstruction. Non-urgent indications for surgery include scenarios in which endoscopic removal is challenging such as trichobezoars [24], or if the object has failed to progress along the GIT and is not accessible by endoscopy [25–27].

Access in all cases is through an upper midline incision. The abdominal wound is also protected to minimize the risk of wound infection. Subsequent surgical removal of gastric

http://dx.doi.org/10.5772/63464

foreign bodies will involve a transverse gastrotomy away from the pylorus and between the lesser and greater curve of the stomach (**Figure 1**).

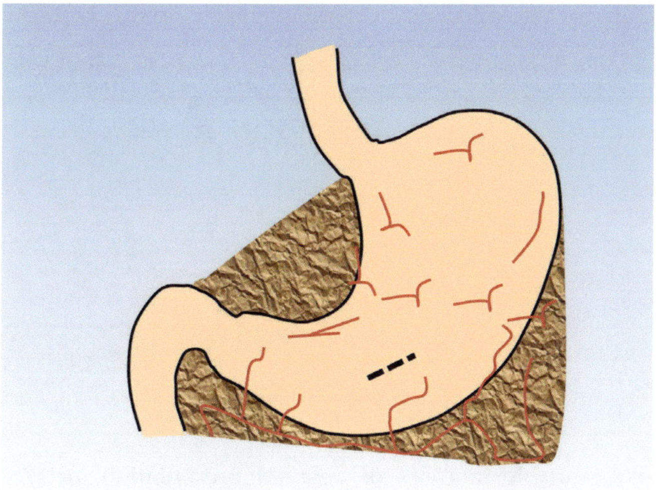

Figure 1. Transverse gastrotomy for removal of foreign bodies.

Objects impacted at the duodenal sweep can be removed through a duodenotomy if they cannot be milked back to the stomach. Similarly, impacted objects in the small bowel can be removed through enterotomies. Primary closure is indicated in cases without peritoneal contamination. For closure, it is important to avoid narrowing the lumen. Techniques similar to that of pyloroplasty involving transverse incisions with longitudinal closure using absorbable sutures should be considered (**Figure 2**).

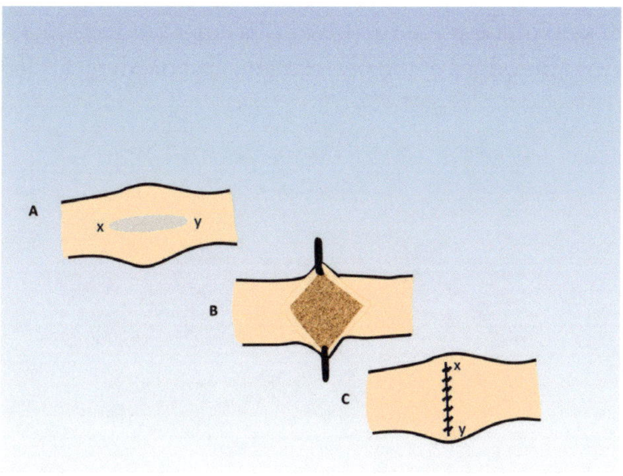

Figure 2. Technique of pyloroplasty.

Perforated cases are often contained, so a primary closure or segmental resection of the affected small bowel may still be possible provided the tissues remain healthy (**Figure 3**).

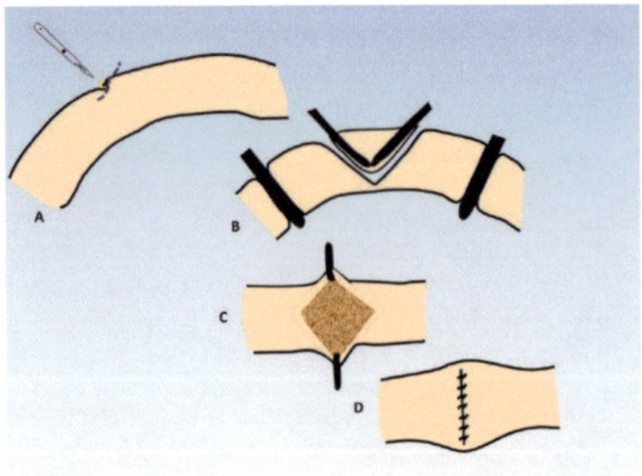

Figure 3. Segmental bowel resection and anastomosis.

Diversion may be reasonable in cases of delayed presentation, or where grossly faecal contamination has occurred, and the tissues are unhealthy. The stoma can be reversed at a later date (after 3 months usually). The use of intra-abdominal drains may be limited to the surgeon's preference. Postoperative care should follow the lines of enhanced recovery following upper gastrointestinal surgery.

Although sealed perforation involving degradable food matter can be treated non-surgically in the initial instance, such a policy requires careful interval assessment by an experienced surgeon with a low threshold for performing laparotomies if clinical improvement is not apparent both to confirm the diagnosis and oversew an unsealed perforation [28]. In most cases, however, the treatment of choice for patients with perforation of the duodenum is laparotomy, peritoneal lavage and simple closure of perforation, usually by omental patch repair [23]. The initial step of the repair involves placement of full-thickness bites at approximately 0.5 cm away from the edges of the perforation, and the defect is left untied (**Figure 4A**).

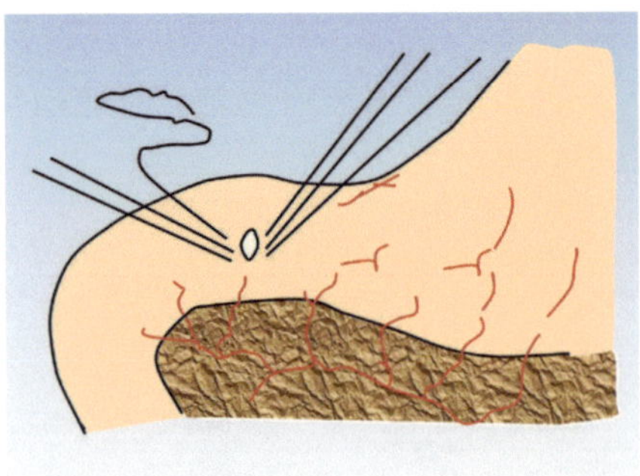

Figure 4A. Placement of sutures for omental patch repair.

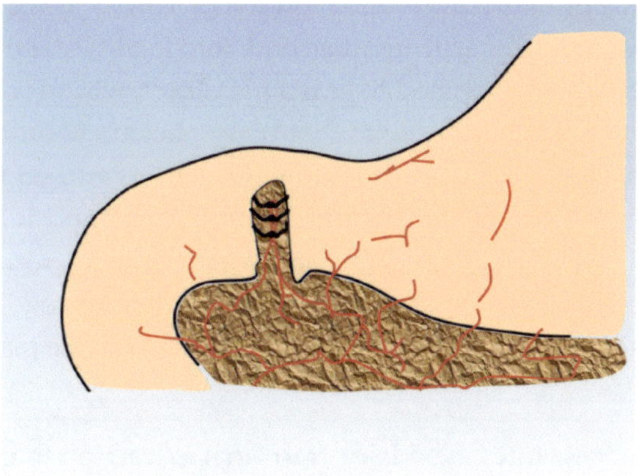

Figure 4B. Final repair of a duodenal perforation with an omental patch.

A patch of omentum is then brought without tension and positioned over the perforation, and the sutures are successively tied to secure the omentum onto the defect itself (**Figure 4B**).

In cases of "giant" perforation, where the defect measures 2.5 cm or more, partial gastrectomy with closure of the duodenal stump should be considered [23]. Alternatively, in situations where the clinical situation or expertise dictates more expeditious surgery, the duodenal perforation should be closed as well as possible around a large Foley or T-tube catheter to create a controlled fistula [23]. Other methods described include a free omental and jejunal serosal "plug" [23].

7.2. Inserted foreign objects and anorectal objects

It is essential to remove all retained anorectal foreign bodies [8]. However, extraction of rectal foreign bodies may be challenging. The medical literature confirms the diversity of the problem, and equally some ingenious solutions [19, 29–40]. Techniques described range from simple digital extraction to complicated surgical removal. Several algorithms for management have also been proposed [6, 7, 29], with a tendency to progress from least to most invasive as required [7]. This approach will result in the best chance of success with the lowest risk to the patient [7].

Unless signs of peritonitis are present, or the patient is unstable, both of which necessitate emergency laparotomy, an initial attempt at bedside extraction is advised [15]. Bedside extraction is successful in 60–75% of cases [7]. A variety of tools can be used as adjunct retrieval devices including obstetric forceps, ring forceps, Kocher clamps, suction devices and various grasping forceps. The instruments used vary according to the characteristics of each case. For example, in cases where the rectal foreign body has created a seal with the rectal mucosa [15], a balloon catheter such as a Foley may be used to pull the foreign body distally along the GIT [41–44]. The Foley is inserted, deflated and passed proximally to the retained object, then inflated and subsequently pulled to drag the foreign body along the bowel. This technique is useful in cases in which the rectal lumen is obstructed by a smooth foreign body. The foreign body results in a negative pressure differential on the proximal rectal lumen. By inserting the Foley above the area, the pressures will equalize and help facilitate the removal. Alternatively, obstetric vacuum extractors may be used to grasp the object, widen the anal canal and release the rectal seal [45–47]. It is pertinent to note that body packers should have potentially toxic packages removed with digital rectal examination only, tools and endoscopic devices should be avoided as they increase the risk of damage to the parcel and leakage/absorption of its' contents. Any systemic signs of perforation may warrant laparotomy with the subsequent supportive care of any overdose geared towards the drug ingested. The use of enemas and stimulants to propel the object distally is not recommended, as these may cause further damage to the rectal wall [7].

Surgeons have higher success rates at bedside transanal extraction than emergency physicians [48]. The exact reasons for this are unclear, but may represent a willingness to be more aggressive in attempts to remove the object and due to the ability to fix resultant damage in the theatre [7]. In general, predictors of failure of transanal extraction of retained rectal foreign bodies include objects longer than 10 cm, hard or sharp objects, those that have migrated into the sigmoid colon as well as those that have been retained for more than 2 days [6, 48].

When attempting to remove a rectal foreign body transanally, the most important factor in successful extraction is patient relaxation [15]. This can be achieved with a perineal nerve block, a spinal anaesthetic or either of these in combination with intravenous conscious sedation [15]. After the patient has been appropriately sedated and anaesthetized, attempts should be made to remove the object [15]. The high lithotomy position in Candy Care Stirrups in the operating theatre facilitates the removal of most objects and has the added benefit of allowing for downwards abdominal pressure to be applied to aid in the extraction of a foreign body [15]. The anal canal should be gently dilated to three fingers' breadth before transanal delivery [15]. A reverse Trendelenburg angulation may also be attempted. The technique of bimanual extraction helps move an object caudally and also prevents cephalad migration with difficult to grasp objects [7]. Blind insertion of instruments should be avoided as it can hinder the removal of the foreign body and induce rectal injuries or perforation [49].

Flexible sigmoidoscopy is required for objects that are located more proximally in the rectum or the distal sigmoid colon, which are often not amenable to removal by per digital rectal examination or with the tools mentioned earlier [29]. Endoscopy produces an additional means of non-operative extraction, thereby limiting operative intervention in some cases. Removal of sharp objects can pose an extra risk to both the patient and the surgeon, but direct visualization with rigid or a flexible endoscopy has helped to mitigate this problem [9, 15]. This excellent visualization of the mucosa with endoscopy also helps to evaluate for subtle and gross changes in the rectal mucosa [15]. Polypectomy snares may be used to "lasso" objects [18, 50] or objects may be grasped by grasping forceps using endoscopic methods. Removal under general anaesthesia is attempted when endoscopic removal under sedation is not successful. It is worth mentioning that all patients undergoing removal of foreign objects under general anaesthesia should also consent for laparoscopy or laparotomy should the first attempts fail [29].

http://dx.doi.org/10.5772/63464

Surgical removal (laparotomy or laparoscopy) is indicated in patients with systemic signs or radiological evidence of perforation. Additionally, surgery may also be performed as a last resort when anal dilatation, manual or forceps extraction have failed to remove the foreign body [29]. The surgical options for a failed transanal extraction vary from minimally invasive techniques to open surgery. Evidence for use of each technique is limited to case series and reports. For the laparoscopic-assisted techniques of removal, the object is milked inferiorly with direct intra-abdominal visualization using a laparoscope and grasper that aids in the eventual transanal extraction [51]. Similarly, a lower midline mini-laparotomy may be used to squeeze the rectum directly and allow transanal removal [52]. Ultimately, if these attempts remain unsuccessful, a colotomy with transabdominal removal can be performed [7]. This is also the technique usually required in an emergent setting where perforation has occurred [7]. If gross contamination or spillage is present, a Hartmann procedure may be the prudent option [7]. However, if tissue quality is good, a primary repair or short segment resection may be performed, and the repair is tested for a leak using protoscopy [8]. This approach is well supported in the trauma literature with experience of blunt and penetrating trauma [7]. Further, the evidence from trauma literature shows that severe faecal contamination, transfusion of more than three units of blood, and single-agent antibiotic prophylaxis are independent factors for abdominal complications following surgery for colorectal trauma [53].

Further notes on the management of rectal perforation are presented here. When patients present with a rectal perforation, they should, at first, be stabilized as with any trauma patient [15]. After stabilization, management depends on three factors: first, whether the patient is clinically stable or unstable, second, whether the perforation is in an intraperitoneal or extraperitoneal location, and last, whether there is significant fecal soilage or not [15]. Preoperative CT scan is required. A well-established order for the management of a rectal perforation secondary to a foreign body is diversion, debridement, distal washout and drainage [15]. Unstable patients, those with multiple comorbidities, those with significant tissue damage and those with delayed presentation more often require a diversion [15]. On the other hand, a primary repair and washout is suited for patients who present early, those with minimal tissue damage and those with little to no contamination [15]. Small extraperitoneal injuries can be managed with observation, avoidance of enteral feeding and antibiotics [15]. However, laparoscopic approach has been successfully applied in the treatment of colonic perforations, and operative outcomes are similar to open procedures in selected patients [15]. In cases of rectal perforation secondary to foreign body insertion, the operator must be aware of the possibility of secondary or occult organ injury. The small bowel, uterus, bladder and sigmoid colon should all be assessed preoperatively. It is also important that a full consent process outlining risk of a stoma is discussed before the patient is anaesthetized. Failure to do so may result in patient dissatisfaction with treatment and complaints.

If none of the above measures are successful, specifically in cases of large objects tightly wedged in the pelvis, the next logical step would be to carry out a symphysiotomy [8]. A symphysiotomy involves attempts at expanding the pelvic volume to facilitate the passage/ removal of larger objects. Such a description may, however, be a historical anecdote rather than acceptable correct surgical practice.

8. Aftercare

If the ingested foreign bodies are not or cannot be removed, a case-by-case approach depending on the size and type of the foreign body is suggested [12]. A patient may be discharged if a successful and uncomplicated endoscopic removal of ingested foreign bodies has been achieved [12]. Other groups of patients including those with significant co-morbidities, delayed presentation, difficult extraction or haemodynamically unstable post-extraction may require further clinical observation. Post-extraction repeat endoscopy and plain radiographs should be considered before discharging any such patient [18, 48].

Psychological evaluation before discharge should be considered in the setting of intentional ingestion. This assessment may help reduce recurrent presentations. In cases of sexual assault, long-term psychological consequences may occur, and therefore, early involvement of mental health services and counselling is warranted [6]. Children in whom a non-accidental injury is suspected should be referred to a paediatrician for further evaluation, and legal authorities should always be informed in every case of suspected assault [6]. The aim is to offer support to victims of assault and abuse [18, 54]. Additionally, the patients should be examined for the use of alcohol and narcotic drugs.

Postoperative pain control, early ambulation and diet initiation upon return of bowel function should follow guidelines for any general surgical intervention [8]. For patients who underwent surgical extraction, the discharge should be considered when bowel physiology returns [8]. For anorectal foreign bodies, it is of paramount importance to inspect the distal colon endoscopically to out rule any unintentional injuries upon successful extraction [10, 18]. It is also important to document sphincter function post-extraction [7]. Although bleeding lacerations in the rectal mucosa are self-limiting, perforation resulting in sepsis and multisystem organ failure can occur [15]. If there is any clinical suspicion, a CT scan with rectal contrast or rectal enema with water-soluble contrast can detect this potentially life-threatening complication [7]. After diagnosis, stable patients may be managed with antibiotics [7]. Patients with signs of toxicity including fever, hypotension or severe pain should be managed by surgical exploration [7]. Depending on the level of perforation, options for surgical management are similar to those previously described above [7].

Significant trauma or damage to the anal sphincter can also result in mild to severe faecal incontinence. There are no good long-term studies, and few articles describe long-term follow-up [7]. One series included a telephone survey of 30 patients with a previous retained foreign body. None had any incontinence to solid, liquid or gas with a follow-up ranging from 8 to 96 months [55]. Although uncommon, complications from sphincter damage may include fistulas and stenosis [56]. Cases of sphincter dysfunction (including incontinence) are often initially managed conservatively; any injury is left open, and further assessment is undertaken in an elective setting [7]. A follow-up of at least 3 months is recommended before considering any sphincter repair [17]. If symptoms persist, a delayed sphincteroplasty may be performed with good results [57].

9. Summary

In keeping with the inquisitive nature of humans, there are a wide variety of foreign body presentations encountered in clinical practice across all age groups. Although there may be anecdotal or interesting clinical scenarios of ingested or inserted foreign bodies, one can never underestimate that there is a significant morbidity and unfortunately, mortality associated with these cases. The retrieval of upper gastrointestinal foreign bodies is a more described pathway in the literature. The removal of rectal foreign bodies often requires a wide variety of approaches, many of which are individualized. Surgery may be necessary in some patients.

10. Suggested additional reading

Birk M, et al. Removal of foreign bodies in the upper gastrointestinal tract in adults: European Society of Gastrointestinal Endoscopy (ESGE) Clinical Guideline. Endoscopy. 2016;48:1-8. https://www.thieme-connect.com/products/ejournals/html/10.1055/s-0042-100456.

Key points

- Presentations due to gastrointestinal foreign body ingestion or insertions are common emergency clinical scenarios. The majority of these objects will pass spontaneously, and others will require endoscopic or surgical intervention for removal.
- Absolute indications for abdominal surgery include those patients with clinical peritonitis from perforation. Other indications for surgery include bowel obstruction and failure of conservative or endoscopic management.
- Surgical technique for removal of a gastric foreign body involves a transverse gastrotomy with incision away from pylorus and between the lesser and greater curvature of the stomach. Retained intestinal or colonic foreign bodies may also be removed through enterotomies or colostomies. Primary closure is indicated in the absence of peritoneal contamination, and it is important to avoid narrowing the gut lumen during closure.
- In the case of peritonitis due to gut perforation, a primary repair or short segment resection of enterotomy or colotomy may be appropriate after a thorough washout of the abdomen if the tissue quality is good. Diversion of the gut may be required in cases of delayed presentations, significant faecal contamination and signs of sepsis.
- Foreign body insertions represent a challenging and unique field of colorectal trauma. A careful history and examination is essential in the diagnosis. However, rectal examination may best be performed after an abdominal X-ray to prevent inadvertent, accidental injury to the surgeon from sharp objects.
- Bimanual extraction under anaesthesia is the technique of first choice when bedside extraction fails. Other options for removal under anaesthesia will include anal dilatation,

laparotomy or laparoscopy. A colotomy may be required for removal when the object cannot be milked down for transanal extraction. A Hartmann's procedure may be necessary in cases of significant faecal peritonitis.

- It is important to document sphincter function post-extraction of a rectal foreign body. Recto-sigmoidoscopy is advised to assess the rectal and distal colonic mucosa to determine the extent of any possible injury and exclude perforation.
- Cases of sphincter dysfunction after removal of a rectal foreign body are often initially managed conservatively, and the majority will resolve without any intervention. For those not settling, referral to a specialized colorectal surgery/incontinence unit is recommended and may require a delayed sphincteroplasty.

Author details

Obinna Obinwa*, David Cooper, James M. O'Riordan and Paul Neary

*Address all correspondence to: obinnaobinwa@rcsi.ie

Department of Surgery, The Adelaide and Meath Hospital, Dublin Incorporating the National Children's Hospital, Dublin, Ireland

References

[1] Pfau PR. Removal and management of esophageal foreign bodies. Techniques in Gastrointestinal Endoscopy. 2014;16(1):32–9.

[2] Lyons MF, 2nd and Tsuchida AM. Foreign bodies of the gastrointestinal tract. The Medical Clinics of North America. 1993;77(5):1101–14.

[3] Clerf LH. Historical aspects of foreign bodies in the air and food passages. Southern Medical Journal. 1975;68(11):1449–54.

[4] Ikenberry SO, Jue TL, Anderson MA, et al. Management of ingested foreign bodies and food impactions. Gastrointestinal Endoscopy. 2011;73(6):1085–91. DOI:10.1016/j.gie.2010.11.010.

[5] Erbil B, Karaca MA, Aslaner MA, et al. Emergency admissions due to swallowed foreign bodies in adults. World Journal of Gastroenterology. 2013;19(38):6447–52. DOI: 10.3748/wjg.v19.i38.6447.

[6] Ayantunde AA. Approach to the diagnosis and management of retained rectal foreign bodies: clinical update. Techniques in Coloproctology. 2013;17(1):13–20. DOI:10.1007/s10151-012-0899-1.

[7] Cologne KG and Ault GT. Rectal foreign bodies: what is the current standard? Clinics in Colon and Rectal Surgery. 2012;25(4):214–8. DOI:10.1055/s-0032-1329392.

[8] Kasotakis G, Roediger L and Mittal S. Rectal foreign bodies: a case report and review of the literature. International Journal of Surgery Case Reports. 2012;3(3):111–5. DOI: 10.1016/j.ijscr.2011.11.007.

[9] Clarke DL, Buccimazza I, Anderson FA, et al. Colorectal foreign bodies. Colorectal Disease: The Official Journal of the Association of Coloproctology of Great Britain and Ireland. 2005;7(1):98–103. DOI:10.1111/j.1463-1318.2004.00699.x.

[10] Akhtar MA and Arora PK. Case of unusual foreign body in the rectum. Saudi Journal of Gastroenterology: Official Journal of the Saudi Gastroenterology Association. 2009;15(2):131–2. DOI:10.4103/1319-3767.48973.

[11] Carp L. Foreign bodies in the intestine. Annals of Surgery. 1927;85(4):575–91.

[12] Birk M, Bauerfeind P, Deprez PH, et al. Removal of foreign bodies in the upper gastrointestinal tract in adults: European Society of Gastrointestinal Endoscopy (ESGE) Clinical Guideline. Endoscopy. 2016;48:1–8. DOI:10.1055/s-0042-100456.

[13] Butterworth J and Feltis B. Toy magnet ingestion in children: revising the algorithm. Journal of Pediatric Surgery. 2007;42(12):e3–5.

[14] Control CfD and Prevention. Gastrointestinal injuries from magnet ingestion in children—United States, 2003–2006. Morbidity and Mortality Weekly Report. 2006;55(48):1296–1300.

[15] Coskun A, Erkan N, Yakan S, et al. Management of rectal foreign bodies. World Journal of Emergency Surgery. 2013;8(1):11. DOI:10.1186/1749-7922-8-11.

[16] Lancashire MJ, Legg PK, Lowe M, et al. Surgical aspects of international drug smuggling. British Medical Journal. 1988;296(6628):1035–7.

[17] Kurer MA, Davey C, Khan S, et al. Colorectal foreign bodies: a systematic review. Colorectal Disease: The Official Journal of the Association of Coloproctology of Great Britain and Ireland. 2010;12(9):851–61. DOI:10.1111/j.1463-1318.2009.02109.x.

[18] Goldberg JE and Steele SR. Rectal foreign bodies. The Surgical Clinics of North America. 2010;90(1):173–84. DOI:10.1016/j.suc.2009.10.004.

[19] Losanoff JE and Kjossev KT. Rectal "oven mitt": the importance of considering a serious underlying injury. The Journal of Emergency Medicine. 1999;17(1):31–3.

[20] Ambe P, Weber SA, Schauer M, et al. Swallowed foreign bodies in adults. Deutsches Arzteblatt International. 2012;109(50):869–75. DOI:10.3238/arztebl.2012.0869.

[21] Ridder GJ, Maier W, Kinzer S, et al. Descending necrotizing mediastinitis: contemporary trends in etiology, diagnosis, management, and outcome. Annals of Surgery. 2010;251(3):528–34. DOI:10.1097/SLA.0b013e3181c1b0d1.

[22] Goh BK, Chow PK, Quah HM, et al. Perforation of the gastrointestinal tract secondary to ingestion of foreign bodies. World Journal of Surgery. 2006;30(3):372–7. DOI:10.1007/s00268-005-0490-2.

[23] Wayman J. Benign ulceration of the stomach and duodenum and the complications of previous ulcer surgery. In: Michael Griffin S, Raimes SA, Shenfine J, editors. Oesophagogastric Surgery: Companion to Specialist Surgical Practice. 5th ed. China: Elsevier; 2014. p. 317–35.

[24] Iwamuro M, Tanaka S, Shiode J, et al. Clinical characteristics and treatment outcomes of nineteen Japanese patients with gastrointestinal bezoars. Internal Medicine. 2014;53(11):1099–105.

[25] Webb WA. Management of foreign bodies of the upper gastrointestinal tract: update. Gastrointestinal Endoscopy. 1995;41(1):39–51.

[26] Ginsberg GG. Management of ingested foreign objects and food bolus impactions. Gastrointestinal Endoscopy. 1995;41(1):33–8.

[27] Smith MT and Wong RK. Foreign bodies. Gastrointestinal Endoscopy Clinics of North America. 2007;17(2):361–82, vii. DOI:10.1016/j.giec.2007.03.002.

[28] Donovan AJ, Berne TV and Donovan JA. Perforated duodenal ulcer: an alternative therapeutic plan. Archives of Surgery. 1998;133(11):1166–71.

[29] Koornstra JJ and Weersma RK. Management of rectal foreign bodies: description of a new technique and clinical practice guidelines. World Journal of Gastroenterology. 2008;14(27):4403–6.

[30] Obinwa O, Robertson I and Stokes M. Removal of a sex toy under general anaesthesia using a bimanual-technique and Magill's forceps: a case report. International Journal of Surgery Case Reports. 2015;15:96–8. DOI:10.1016/j.ijscr.2015.08.014.

[31] Couch CJ, Tan EG and Watt AG. Rectal foreign bodies. The Medical Journal of Australia. 1986;144(10):512–5.

[32] Graves RW, Allison EJ, Jr., Bass RR, et al. Anal eroticism: two unusual rectal foreign bodies and their removal. Southern Medical Journal. 1983;76(5):677–8.

[33] Siroospour D and Dragstedt LR, 2nd. A large foreign body removed through the intact anus: report of a case. Diseases of the Colon and Rectum. 1975;18(7):616–9.

[34] Ahmed A and Cummings SA. Novel endoscopic approach for removal of a rectal foreign body. Gastrointestinal Endoscopy. 1999;50(6):872–4.

[35] Glaser J, Hack T and Rubsam M. Unusual rectal foreign body: treatment using argon-beam coagulation. Endoscopy. 1997;29(3):230–1. DOI:10.1055/s-2007-1004178.

[36] Wolf L and Geraci K. Colonscopic removal of balloons from the bowel. Gastrointestinal Endoscopy. 1977;24(1):41.

[37] Peet TN. Removal of impacted rectal foreign body with obstetric forceps. British Medical Journal. 1976;1(6008):500–1.

[38] Aquino MM and Turner JW. A simple technique for removing an impacted aerosol-can cap from the rectum. Diseases of the Colon and Rectum. 1986;29(10):675.

[39] Clark SK and Karanjia ND. A cork in a bottle—a simple technique for removal of a rectal foreign body. Annals of the Royal College of Surgeons of England. 2003;85(4): 282.

[40] Hughes JP, Marice HP and Gathright JB, Jr. Method of removing a hollow object from the rectum. Diseases of the Colon and Rectum. 1976;19(1):44–5.

[41] Manimaran N, Shorafa M and Eccersley J. Blow as well as pull: an innovative technique for dealing with a rectal foreign body. Colorectal Disease: The Official Journal of the Association of Coloproctology of Great Britain and Ireland. 2009;11(3):325–6. DOI: 10.1111/j.1463-1318.2008.01653.x.

[42] Safioleas M, Stamatakos M, Safioleas C, et al. The management of patients with retained foreign bodies in the rectum: from surgeon with respect. Acta Chirurgica Belgica. 2009;109(3):352–5.

[43] Yaman M, Deitel M, Burul CJ, et al. Foreign bodies in the rectum. Canadian Journal of Surgery. Journal Canadien de Chirurgie. 1993;36(2):173–7.

[44] Diwan VS. Removal of 100-watt electric bulb from rectum. Annals of Emergency Medicine. 1982;11(11):643–4.

[45] Feigelson S, Maun D, Silverberg D, et al. Removal of a large spherical foreign object from the rectum using an obstetric vacuum device: a case report. The American Surgeon. 2007;73(3):304–6.

[46] Johnson SO and Hartranft TH. Nonsurgical removal of a rectal foreign body using a vacuum extractor. Report of a case. Diseases of the Colon and Rectum. 1996;39(8):935–7.

[47] Mackinnon RP. Removing rectal foreign bodies: is the ventouse gender specific? The Medical Journal of Australia. 1998;169(11–12):670–1.

[48] Lake JP, Essani R, Petrone P, et al. Management of retained colorectal foreign bodies: predictors of operative intervention. Diseases of the Colon and Rectum. 2004;47(10): 1694–8.

[49] Lim KJ, Kim JS, Kim BG, et al. Removal of rectal foreign bodies using tenaculum forceps under endoscopic assistance. Intestinal Research. 2015;13(4):355-9. DOI:10.5217/ir. 2015.13.4.355.

[50] Singaporewalla RM, Tan DE and Tan TK. Use of endoscopic snare to extract a large rectosigmoid foreign body with review of literature. Surgical Laparoscopy, Endoscopy & Percutaneous Techniques. 2007;17(2):145–8. DOI:10.1097/SLE.0b013e318045bf1a.

[51] Berghoff KR and Franklin ME, Jr. Laparoscopic-assisted rectal foreign body removal: report of a case. Diseases of the Colon and Rectum. 2005;48(10):1975–7. DOI:10.1007/s10350-005-0117-6.

[52] Yildiz SY, Kendirci M, Akbulut S, et al. Colorectal emergencies associated with penetrating or retained foreign bodies. World Journal of Emergency Surgery. 2013;8(1): 25. DOI:10.1186/1749-7922-8-25.

[53] Demetriades D, Murray JA, Chan L, et al. Penetrating colon injuries requiring resection: diversion or primary anastomosis? An AAST prospective multicenter study. The Journal of Trauma. 2001;50(5):765–75.

[54] Huang WC, Jiang JK, Wang HS, et al. Retained rectal foreign bodies. Journal of the Chinese Medical Association. 2003;66(10):607–12.

[55] Ooi BS, Ho YH, Eu KW, et al. Management of anorectal foreign bodies: a cause of obscure anal pain. The Australian and New Zealand Journal of Surgery. 1998;68(12): 852-5.

[56] Rodriguez-Hermosa JI, Codina-Cazador A, Ruiz B, et al. Management of foreign bodies in the rectum. Colorectal Disease: The Official Journal of the Association of Coloproctology of Great Britain and Ireland. 2007;9(6):543–8. DOI:10.1111/j.1463-1318.2006.01184.x.

[57] Crass RA, Tranbaugh RF, Kudsk KA, et al. Colorectal foreign bodies and perforation. American Journal of Surgery. 1981;142(1):85–8.

Chapter 6

Non-Surgical Causes of Acute Abdominal Pain

Ferdane Sapmaz, Sebahat Başyiğit,
Murat Başaran and Selim Demirci

Additional information is available at the end of the chapter

http://dx.doi.org/10.5772/64176

Abstract

Abdominal pain constitutes 5% of the causes of emergency admissions and is an important part in the practice of emergency services in all centers. Patients may suffer from acute surgical abdomen, acute abdomen with nonsurgical diseases or acute problems of chronic diseases. Abdominal pain is sometimes associated with acute trauma. Clinical assessment is a process where diagnosis and treatment must be done quickly and must be well managed. We have tried here to discuss the non-surgical causes of abdominal pain.

Keywords: Emergency Acute, Abdominal, Pain, Non-surgical, Acute abdomen

1. Introduction

Acute abdomen describes the sudden and severe starting of abdominal pain with unexplained etiology [1]. Case management should be done fairly quickly. Nonsurgical diseases as well as surgical pathologies could be the cause of acute abdomen.

Medical history and physical examination findings are very important for assessment. Abdominal pain is the most important sign of acute abdomen but might not be observed in each cases [2]. Especially the elderly and children should be considered for acute abdomen.

Abdominal pain is usually a feature, but a pain-free acute abdomen can occur, particularly in older people, in children, in the immunocompromised, and in the women during their last trimester of pregnancy. Acute abdominal complaints are common [3].

The differential diagnosis of acute abdomen should be done as soon as possible with the medical history, physical examination, laboratory and radiological findings; and the diagnosis should be accelerated for patient management [4].

2. Pathophysiology

2.1. Visceral pain

Visceral pain is a kind of a pain resulting from abdominal, pelvic and thoracic organs whose mechanism is not clearly understood and thus, very difficult to identify [5]. Visceral pain is a common, often superficial pain which cannot be localized. Nausea, vomiting, and emotional changes can accompany this pain [6].

Visceral pain does not result from every organ and is not always associated with tissue damage. Sensitivity of certain organs to pain depends on the properties of the peripheral receptors of organs [7]. The spread of the visceral pain over a large area depends on the distribution of visceral afferent nociceptive pathways in the central nervous system.

Visceral pain usually occurs as a result of the excessive stress of hollow organs such as the digestive tract, the gall bladder, and the ureter or contraction of smooth muscles [8]. Visceral pain may also occur as a result of the stress of the capsule around the organs such as kidney, liver and spleen. The internal organs do not have parenchyma and pain receptors in the brain. Visceral pain receptors are located where there are artery walls, peritoneum, pleura and dura mater and other connective tissues [9].

2.2. Somatic pain

Somatic pain is a type of nociceptive pain. It is the pain growing in all body zones including the skin, muscles and joints except the internal organs. Arising from the somatic nerves, the pain begins suddenly distinct from the visceral pain and is sharp and well localized.

The somatic pain sensation in the portion below the head comes along with the spinal nerve fibers in the spinal ganglia in the posterior radix [10].

Somatic pain can be either *superficial* or *deep*.

2.2.1. Superficial Somatic Pain

Superficial pain arises from nociceptive receptors in the skin and mucous membranes. For example, if you cut your lip, this pain is called superficial somatic pain. Superficial somatic pain is the type of pain that happens with common everyday injuries and is characterized as pricking, sharp, burning or throbbing pain [11].

2.2.2. Deep Somatic Pain

Deep somatic pain originates from structures deeper in your body, such as joints, bones, tendons and muscles. Like visceral pain, deep somatic pain is usually dull and aching. Deep somatic pain can either be experienced either locally or more generally depending on the degree of trauma. For example, if you bump your knee, then the pain that you experience is local to your knee. However, if you break your kneecap, or patella, you experience pain in your whole leg [12].

2.3. Referred pain

Referred pain is feeling pain in a different region than the area where the abdominal organs affected by the disease are located [13]. Referred pain can be felt in the deeper parts of the skin or tissue and can be well localized. Stress with air or fluid in the intestines can cause this type of pain [14]. It occurs due to the simultaneous arrival of the somatic afferent nerve fibers innervating the dermatome where the referred pain is sensed and the visceral afferent fibers that innervate the affected abdominal organs to the spinal cord. Referred pain sometimes has hyperesthesia along with pain [15].

2.4. Stimuli leading to abdominal pain

Pain-sensing receptors (nociceptors) are located in the muscle layer of hollow organs such as the bowel and in the capsule of the solid organs such as the liver. Intra-abdominal organs (abdominal viscera) and the mesentery are insensitive to stimuli such as cutting, crashing or tearing that can normally evoke pain in the skin [16]. There are three kinds of stimuli that can alert the nociceptors in the abdominal organs: (1) tension or withdrawal of the visceral walls, (2) inflammation (due to chemical mediators and edema arising in the inflammation area such as bradykinin, serotonin, leukotrienes and prostaglandins) and (3) ischemia (due to the accumulation of metabolites and chemical mediators in the tissues). Visceral peritoneum (serosa), liver parenchyma and greater omentum are insensitive to pain [17]. Inflammation caused by chemicals and bacteria in the parietal peritoneum is an important cause of pain. Inflammation and edema in the tissues lower pain threshold. The other two important reasons for abdominal pain are the stress of the neoplastic formations or fibrotic tissues on the nerve roots [18, 19].

3. Non-surgical disorders causing acute abdominal pain

Abdominal pain is the most constant symptom of acute abdomen whether of surgical or non-surgical origin. Non-surgical causes of acute abdominal pain stimulating an acute abdomen account for up to 30% of patients requiring hospital admission [20].

The history and physical examination remain the critical first step in effective management and must be based on a thorough understanding of the anatomy and physiology of abdominal pain. Laboratory studies are of limited value. Complete blood count (CBC), urinalysis, serum lipase and pregnancy test are most helpful, particularly when abnormal.

Computed tomography (CT) has led to the greatest improvement in the care of patients with acute abdominal pain. Its value for any given patient depends on a given institution's experience in its application and interpretation.

3.1. Metabolic/endocrine causes

3.1.1. Diabetic ketoacidosis

Diabetic ketoacidosis (DKA) and hyperosmolar hyperglycemic state (HHS) are among the most serious and accurate metabolic complications of diabetes [21]. These situations can be observed in both type 1 and type 2 diabetes mellitus (DM). While the mortality rate is below 5% in good hands in diabetic ketoacidosis (DKA), it is at a level as high as 15% in hyperosmolar hyperglycemic state (HHS). In both cases, the prognosis worsens with aging in the presence of coma and hypertension. Fifteen percent to 67% of type 1 diabetic patients have DKA in the first diagnosis [22]. Absolute or partial insulin deficiency is the underlying reason in metabolic disorders in DKA. The consequences of insulin deficiency become more pronounced with the strong impact of catecholamines, glucagon, cortisol and counterregulatory hormones (anti-insulin hormones). As a result, glucose production by the liver and kidney increases and finally hyperglycemia and hyperosmolarity occur. Increasing lipolysis and ketone bodies production causes ketosis and acidosis [23]. Hyperglycemia and acidosis result in osmotic diuresis, dehydration and the loss of essential electrolytes.

Polyuria, polydipsia, polyphagia history, weight loss, vomiting, abdominal pain, dehydration, weakness, confusion and as a result coma are the classical clinical observations of DKA.

Abdominal pain can mimic acute abdomen especially in children. The abdominal complaints can be seen in 40%–75% of the patients with DKA [24].

There have been many studies on the mechanism of abdominal pain in DKA; however, a complete mechanism has not been established. It was observed that after hyperglycemia, ketoacidosis and dehydration are improved, especially abdominal pain complaints disappeared. In some DKA cases, it was reported that exploratory laparotomy was applied due to the problem of diagnosis and it was associated with high morbidity and mortality [25].

Diabetic ketoacidosis	High serum glucose
Familial Mediterranean fever	Pleuritis, peritonitis
Porphyria	High porphobilinogen
Addison disease	Low serum cortisol
Hyperthyroidism	Low TSH
Hypokalemia	Low serum potassium
Hypophosphatemia	Low serum phosphate
Hypercalcemia	High serum calcium

Table 1. Metabolic causes.

The possibility of abdomen surgery should always be kept in mind in the cases where abdominal complaints do not disappear despite DKA treatment.

Abdominal pain in DKA might be correlated with the weight of metabolic acidosis and might be confused with an acute abdominal crisis. Other metabolic causes are listed in **Table 1**.

3.2. Hematologic/immunological causes

3.2.1. Sickle cell crisis

Sickle cell anemia (SCA) is a genetic disorder caused by abnormal hemoglobin S production. Hemoglobin S is formed by replacing the glutamic acid in 6th stage of the beta chain with valine. SCA is characterized by recurrent vaso-occlusive crisis [26]. Vaso-occlusive crisis is an emergency that requires frequent hospitalization of the patients with SCA [27]. Although pathophysiology and treatment of various crises are known, mortality rate associated with this disease is high. The mortality rate in this disease is the highest in the first 5 years of life. Almost half of these mortalities occur in the second 6 months of life. Acute infections and serious anemic sequestrations are the most common causes of death [28].

Sickle-shaped erythrocytes reduce the flow of circulation and the blood flow slows down. This leads to congestion especially in the small vessels and creates an anaerobic environment. Some of the sickle cells are recycled and can take their normal form. However, some others cannot go back to their normal form due to the permanent destruction occurring in their cell membranes. These cells lead to hypoxia in the tissues, leading to atherosclerosis and cause painful crisis and organ necrosis as well as tissue damage in the acute and chronic processes.

Vaso-occlusive, in other words, painful crises are usually the first symptom of the disease and are the most common complication after the newborn period [29]. Initiating factors in acute painful episodes may be exposure to cold, dehydration, infection, stress, menstruation or alcohol intake. The initiator cause is infection in 80% of patients [30].

Sickle cell crisis	Sickle cells, effusions
Thrombotic thrombocytopenic purpura	Thrombocytopenia, fever, confusion
Hemolytic uremic syndrome	Schistocytes on smear
Food allergy	Increased Ig E level
Henoch-Schönlein purpura	Leukocytoclastic vasculitis with Ig A deposition
Mast cell activation syndrome	Serologic markers as above
Hereditary angioneurotic edema	Low C1 esterase inhibitor level

Table 2. Hematologic/immunologic causes.

Intravascular sickling causes blockages in small blood vessels and eventually internal organs and soft tissue necrosis [31]. Necrosis shows itself with common bone, joint and muscle pain. Although pain may affect any area of the body, back, chest, abdomen and extremities are most commonly affected. The severity of the pain can be too light that can be ignored or too severe to be tolerated. Findings such as fever, joint swelling, tenderness, tachypnea, hypertension, nausea and vomiting may accompany painful crisis [32].

Widespread and persistent abdominal pain is one of the most common complaints. It can be difficult to distinguish abdominal pain from abdominal events, such as sickle cell crises, cholecystitis and appendicitis. Patients might be aware of the difference or similarities of the pain with the previous episodes and can distinguish it. There should not be peritonitis symptoms such as rebound tenderness in the abdominal examination of patients with typical vaso-occlusive episodes. This finding is important to distinguish from other diseases that cause acute abdomen.

Other hematologic and immunologic causes are listed in **Table 2**.

3.3. Cardiopulmonary/vascular causes

3.3.1. Myocardial infarction

One of the pathologies that comes to mind foremost in patients presenting acute abdominal pain is acute coronary syndrome. The symptoms of acute myocardial infarction are not always typical. Symptoms especially in inferior myocardial infarction can be confused with gastrointestinal (GI) symptoms. Myocardial infarction pain is very severe and is often described by patients as unbearable. The time is long and often over 30 minutes. It can last for hours. Associated symptoms such as nausea, vomiting and sweating can be seen in approximately half of the cases [33].

Electrocardiogram (ECG) in differentiating the causes of abdominal pain is therefore a very important move. However, although half of the patients experience acute coronary syndrome, it should be noted that the ECG can be negative. In this case, the serum levels of cardiac markers are important for the diagnosis.

Cardiac troponin I (cTnI) is a key protein in cardiac muscle contraction and relaxation. Three to six hours after the start of the acute myocardial infarction (AMI), cTnI release from necrotic myocardium starts and peaks in 24–48 hours. It stays high for 10 days after the initiation of AMI. It is a perfect and specific, long-term, high-residual marker for AMI. In particular, in unstable angina and non-Q wave AMI, detection of elevated serum cTnI level while serum creatine kinase-MB (CK-MB) levels are in the normal range indicates that cTnI is highly sensitive for minimal myocardial damage [34].

Myocardial infarction	Abnormal ECG, high troponin
Aortic dissection	Diagnostic CT angiogram
Pulmonary embolus	High D-dimer diagnostic CT angiography
Pneumonia	Chest radiograph

Table 3. Cardiopulmonary/vascular causes.

No classic findings in the beginning of AMI and frequent complaints of abdominal pain may present various clinical cases that may delay early and accurate diagnosis [35].

Other cardiopulmonary or vascular causes are listed in **Table 3**.

3.4. Infectious causes

3.4.1. Malaria

Malaria is a parasite infection formed by protozoa from the plasmodium family and transmitted to humans by anopheles breed of mosquitoes, which progress with bouts of fever, anemia and splenomegaly, and tends to be initially acute and chronic when left untreated [36]. Malaria agents are *Plasmodium falciparum, Plasmodium vivax, Plasmodium ovale, Plasmodium malaria* and, the newly defined in 2008, *Plasmodium knowlesii.* According to the data obtained from 106 endemic countries where the majority is African countries by the World Health Organization (WHO), about 3.3 billion people faced the risk of malaria in 2010. In 2010, 216 million malaria episodes occurred worldwide, 81% of these were observed in African countries. Because of the infection, 655,000 people died, and the majority of deaths (91%) are still in the African continent. Unfortunately, 86% of the deaths in the world are of children under 5 years of age [37].

Abdominal pain can be traced in malaria due to many reasons. More abdominal symptoms are seen in falciparum malaria when compared to vivax malaria. The abdominal pain is believed to be secondary developing microvascular occlusions to the developing excessive red blood cell sequestration [38].

The pain in malaria cases is usually transient and mild, but in some cases it may be very severe and take longer time to reside. It should be kept in mind that complications such as acalculous cholecystitis, GI bleeding, splenic rupture and splenic infarction may develop in malaria cases [39].

Other infection causes are listed in **Table 4**.

Malaria	Fever, hemolytic anemia, myalgia, multiorgan disease
Staphylotoxin	Fever, rush
Tuberculosis mesenteritis	Fever, diarrhea, ascites
Yersinia enterocolitica	Diarrhea, fever, positive stool culture
Dengue fever	Fever, hemolytic anemia, low platelets

Table 4. Infectious causes.

3.5. Drug/toxin causes

Drugs and toxins can manifest themselves as acute abdominal pain sources through several mechanisms. For example, corrosives can cause acute abdomen by causing serious side effects on the GI tract. Anticholinergic drugs and narcotics may be the cause of partial obstruction of ileus. Again, vasoconstrictor drugs can create acute abdominal pain due to ischemic colitis. Many drugs can cause serious toxic effects especially on the properties of the liver and pancreas, and patients may present with severe acute abdominal symptoms.

Some drugs and toxins are listed in **Table 5**.

Salicylate	Tinnitus, confusion, metabolic acidosis
Tricyclic antidepressants	Anticholinergic symptoms, ECG changes, delirium
Anticholinergics	Tachycardia, confusion, ileus
Heavy metals	Renal, neurologic toxicity
Cocaine	Hypertension, systemic and organ ischemia

Table 5. Drug/toxin causes.

3.6. Neuropsychiatric causes

3.6.1. Herpes zoster

It is the reactivation of zoster latent varicella zoster virus (VZV) infection. VZV that can reside in the sensory nerve ganglia after chickenpox can cause shingles with lesions anatomically similar to those in chicken pox along the dorsal ganglia usually years later [40]. These lesions are controlled with host immune responses (especially, anti-VZV cytotoxic T cells) and recover within a few weeks [41]. Rarely in immune-sufficient people, complications can develop such as very painful, ongoing post-herpetic neuralgia, meningitis, encephalitis, eye involvement, perivasculitis and atypical necrotizing retinopathy [42]. Very severe and life-threatening shingles can be seen in immunocompromised people (suffering from HIV infection and some cancers) [43].

Herpes zoster	Unilateral, painful vesicular rash in dermatomal distribution
Temporal lobe seizures	Aura, abnormal EEG
Radiculopathy	Mechanical pain in dermatomal distribution
Functional abdominal pain syndrome	In woman, fatigue
Abdominal migraine	Adolescent, cyclic occurrence
Irritable bowel syndrome	Diarrhea, constipation

Table 6. Neuropsychiatric causes.

In zona zoster infection, acute abdominal pain is one of the symptoms and may be strong enough to cause laparotomic evaluation by mixing with surgical acute abdominal pain. The reason for 3 of the 121 laparotomies made in a series was found to be zona zoster [44].

A much more acute clinical picture is the abdominal zoster clinic that may occur in the immune-suppressed patients. These patients present dermis findings that progress very commonly within hours and very serious abdominal pain. Especially for these patients, mortality rate is very high despite treatment.

Other neurophsychiatric causes are listed in **Table 6**.

3.7. Renal causes

3.7.1. Nephrolithiasis

It gives similar symptoms to renal and ureteral stones. There are two main symptoms: lumbar pain and hematuria. Lumbar pain may be blunt or renal colic. Pain is felt in the costovertebral angle; it can stay in this area especially during renal colic and it can may spread downwards in the abdomen, groin, genital or femoral region. In addition, complaints such as cold sweats, nausea and vomiting can also be added to the case with increased sympathetic tone. If the infection occurs in the upper urinary tract, symptoms such as fever and pyuria occur in addition to this scene. Fever varies according to the degree of obstruction made by the stone from the remittent fever case to the continuous high fever case.

Other renal causes are listed in **Table 7**.

Nephrolithiasis	Hematuria
Papillary necrosis	Hematuria, diabetes, sickle cell disease

Table 7. Renal causes.

3.8. Vasculitis/connective tissue causes

3.8.1. Systemic lupus erythematosus

Systemic lupus erythematosus (SLE) is a chronic, of unknown cause, connective tissue disease with immunologic disorders and is of autoimmune nature and affects many organs and systems [45]. The disease varies from clinical fever, swelling in the joints, erythematous skin rash to impact on organs and systems, such as kidney, central nervous system and lungs. The majority of patients might have specific organs and system symptoms along with nonspecific systemic symptoms such as weakness and fatigue, fever, muscle aches and weight loss. The disease may sometimes mimic infection starting with fever or may progress in an insidious way in months and years with fever, fatigue and weakness symptoms. Clinical course may range from mild to severe; remission and flare-ups occur typically at varying periods.

Nonspecific gastrointestinal symptoms are seen in lupus patients [46]. Loss of appetite, nausea, vomiting and abdominal pain may develop due to inflammation of the peritoneum (aseptic peritonitis), intestinal vascular disease (mesenteric vasculitis) or drug therapy (NSAIDs and corticosteroids). It may progress to mesentery vasculitis intestinal ischemia, infarction or perforation. The participation of esophagus in the disease is as esophagitis, esophageal ulceration or esophageal motility disorder. Hepatitis and chronic pancreatitis are rare.

Gastrointestinal (GI) manifestations occur in approximately 25–40% of patients with SLE [47]. Many of these symptoms are nonspecific and often reflect either lupus of the GI tract or the effects of medication. Lupus mesenteric vasculitis (LMV) is a predominant cause of acute abdominal pain in SLE patients [48], and it occurs at a high frequency in association with active disease. LMV varies from 29 to 65% among SLE patients with acute abdominal pain. CT is the imaging method of choice to confirm the diagnosis because it permits the visualization of the bowel wall and abdominal vasculature. CT findings include characteristic dilated bowel loops, focal or diffused bowel-wall thickening, abnormal bowel-wall enhancement (target sign), mesenteric edema, stenosis or engorgement of the mesenteric vessels, causing the comb sign and ascites [49, 50]. The CT findings in the present case were consistent with that of acute abdomen because of SLE.

Other connective tissue causes are listed in **Table 8**.

Systemic lupus erythematosus	SLE criteria
Systemic vasculitis	Multiorgan disease with positive p-ANCA
Scleroderma	Skin changes, visceral disease, Scl-70

Table 8. Vasculitis/connective tissue causes.

Author details

Ferdane Sapmaz[1*], Sebahat Başyiğit[1], Murat Başaran[2] and Selim Demirci[3]

*Address all correspondence to: ferda-sapmaz@hotmail.com

1 Kecioren Education and Training Hospital, Department of Gastroenterology, Pınarbaşı, Keçiören, Turkey

2 Yıldırım Beyazıt University of Medicine, Department of Gastroenterology, Çankaya, Turkey

3 Dr. Abdurrahman Yurtaslan Education and Training Hospital, Department of Gastroenterology, Yenimahalle, Turkey

References

[1] Brewer RJ, Golden GT, Hitsch DC, et al. Abdominal pain: an analysis of 1,000 consecutive cases in a university hospital emergency room. Am J Surg 1976; 131:219–224.

[2] Brown FR. The problem of abdominal pain. Br Med J 1942; 1:543.

[3] Fleischer AB Jr, Gardner EF, Feldman SR. Are patients' chief complaints generally specific to one organ system? Am J Manag Care 2001; 7:299.

[4] Yamamoto W, Kono H, Maekawa M, Fukui T. The relationship between abdominal pain regions and specific diseases: an epidemiologic approach to clinical practice. J Epidemiol 1997; 7:27.

[5] Ray BS, Neill CL. Abdominal visceral sensation in man. Ann Surg 1947; 126:709.

[6] Ryle JA. Visceral pain and referred pain. Lancet 1926; 1:895.

[7] Schossmann JM, Holtmann G, Mayer EA. Epidemiology and clinical phenomenology of visceral pain. Schmerz 2002; 16(6):447–451.

[8] Waldmann R. Proton-gated cation channels--neuronal acid sensors in the central and peripheral nervous system. Adv Exp Med Biol 2001; 502:293.

[9] Mannion RJ, Costigan M, Decosterd I, et al. Neurotrophins: peripherally and centrally acting modulators of tactile stimulus-induced inflammatory pain hypersensitivity. Proc Natl Acad Sci U S A 1999; 96:9385.

[10] Classification of chronic pain. Descriptions of chronic pain syndromes and definitions of pain terms. Prepared by the International Association for the Study of Pain, Subcommittee on Taxonomy. Pain Suppl 1986; 3:1.

[11] Bennett M. The LANSS Pain Scale: the Leeds assessment of neuropathic symptoms and signs. Pain 2001; 92:147.

[12] Woolf CJ. Dissecting out mechanisms responsible for peripheral neuropathic pain: implications for diagnosis and therapy. Life Sci 2004; 74:2605.

[13] Arendt-Nielsen L, Svensson P. Referred muscle pain: basic and clinical findings. Clin J Pain 2001; 17(1):11–19.

[14] Witting N, Svensson P, Gottrup H, Arendt-Nielsen L, Jensen TS. Intramuscular and intradermal injection of capsaicin: a comparison of local and referred pain. Pain 2000; 84(2–3):407–412.

[15] Demco LA. Pain referral patterns in the pelvis. J Am Assoc Gynecol Laparosc 2000; 7(2): 181–183.

[16] Worken HJ, Biel FJ, Machella TE. Supradiaphragmatic reference of pain from the colon. Gastroenterology 1952; 22:222.

[17] Arendt-Nielsen L, Svensson P. Referred muscle pain: basic and clinical findings. Clin J Pain 2001; 17(1):11.

[18] Mense S. The pathogenesis of muscle pain. Curr Pain Headache Rep 2003; 7:419–425.

[19] Graven-Nielsen T, Aspegren KS, Henriksson KG, et al. Ketamine reduces muscle pain, temporal summation, and referred pain in fibromyalgia patients. Pain 1999; 85:483–491.

[20] Viniol A, Keunecke C, Biroga T, Stadje R, Dornieden K, Bösner S, Donner-Banzhoff N, Haasenritter J, Becker A. Studies of the symptom abdominal pain--a systematic review and meta-analysis. Fam Pract 2014; 31(5):517–529.

[21] Kitabchi AE, Umpierrez GE, Miles JM, Fisher JN. Hyperglycemic crises in adult patients with diabetes. Diabetes Care 2009; 32(7):1335–1343.

[22] Neufeld ND, Raffel LJ, Landon C, et al. Early presentation of type 2 diabetes in Mexican-American youth. Diabetes Care 1998; 21:80.

[23] Kitabchi AE, Umpierrez GE, Fisher JN, et al. Thirty years of personal experience in hyperglycemic crises: diabetic ketoacidosis and hyperglycemic hyperosmolar state. J Clin Endocrinol Metab 2008; 93:1541.

[24] Sulway MJ, Malins JM. Acetone in diabetic ketoacidosis. Lancet 1970; 2:736.

[25] Loh TP, Saw S, Sethi SK. Bedside monitoring of blood ketone for management of diabetic ketoacidosis: proceed with care. Diabet Med 2012; 29:827.

[26] Embury SH, Hebbel RP, Mohandas N, editors. Sickle Cell Disease. Basic Principles and Clinical Picture. New York: Raven Press; 1994.

[27] Stockman JA, Nigro MA, Mishkin MM, et al. Occlusion of large cerebral vessels in sickle cell anemia. N Engl J Med 1972; 287:846–850.

[28] Charache S, Terrin ML, Moore RD, et al. Effect of hydroxyurea on the frequency of painful crises in sickle cell anemia. N Engl J Med 1995; 332:1317–1322.

[29] Benjamin LJ, Dampier CD, Jacox A, et al. Guideline for the Management of Acute and Chronic Pain in Sickle Cell Disease. Glenview (IL): American Pain Society; 1999.

[30] Benjamin LJ, Swinson GI, Nagel RL. Sickle cell anemia day hospital: an approach for the management of uncomplicated painful crises. Blood 2000; 95:1130–1137.

[31] Ballas SK, Smith ED. Red cell changes during the evolution of the sickle cell painful crisis. Blood 1992; 79:2154–2163.

[32] Milner PF, Kraus AP, Sebes JL, et al. Sickle cell disease as a cause of osteonecrosis of the femoral head. N Engl J Med 1991; 325:1476–1481.

[33] Acute Coronary Syndrome Guidelines Working Group. Guidelines for the management of acute coronary syndromes 2006. Med J Aust 2006; 184:S9–S29.

[34] Ghaemmaghami C, Brady W. Pitfalls in the emergency department diagnosis of acute myocardial infarction. Emerg Med Clin North Am 2001; 19:351–369.

[35] Winters M, Katzen S. Identifying chest pain emergencies in the primary care setting. Prim Care 2006; 33:625–642.

[36] Song HH, O SO, Kim SH, et al. Clinical features of Plasmodium vivax malaria. Korean J Intern Med 2003; 18:220–224.

[37] Taksande A, Vilhekar K, Jain M, Atkari S. Clinico-haematological profile of cerebral malaria in a rural hospital. J Ind Acad Clin Med 2006; 7:308–312.

[38] Kumar A, Taksande AM, Vilhekar KY. Acalculous cholecystitis by P. falciparum in a 3-year-old child. J Vector Borne Dis 2008; 45:76–77.

[39] Mokashi AJ, Shirahatti RG, Prabhu SK, Vagholkar KR. Pathological rupture of malarial spleen. J Postgrad Med 1992; 38:141–142.

[40] Gucuyener K, Citak EC, Elli M, Serdaroglu A, Citak FE. Complications of varicella zoster. Indian J Pediatr. 2002; 69(2):195–196.

[41] Yakushijin Y, Minamoto Y, Takada K, et al. A case of fatal varicella zoster infection with refractory abdominal pain as an early symptom. Kansenshogaku Zasshi 2004; 78(1):64–69.

[42] Kim MK, Strait RT, Sato TT, Hennes HM. A randomized clinical trial of analgesia in children with acute abdominal pain. Acad Emerg Med 2002; 9(4):281–287.

[43] Choo PW, Donahue JG, Manson JE, Plott R. The epidemiology of varicella and its complications. J Infect Dis 1995; 172:706–712.

[44] Rogers SY, Irving W, Harris A, Russell NH. Visceral varicella zoster infection after bone marrow transplantation without skin involvement and the use of PCR for diagnosis. Bone Marrow Transplant 1995; 15:805–807.

[45] Dubois EL, Tuffanelli DL. Clinical manifestations of systemic lupus erythematosus. Computer analysis of 520 cases. JAMA 1964; 190:104–111.

[46] Izbicki JR, Schneider CG, Kastl S. Partial ischemia. Occlusive and nonocclusive mesenteric ischemia, ischemic colitis, systemic lupus erythematosus. Chirurg 2003; 74(5):413–418.

[47] Lee CK, Ahn MS, Lee EY, et al. Acute abdominal pain in systemic lupus erythematosus: focus on lupus enteritis (gastrointestinal vasculitis). Ann Rheum Dis 2002; 61(6):547–550.

[48] Merrill JT. Measuring disease activity in systemic lupus: progress and problems. J Rheumatol. 2002; 29(11):2256–2257.

[49] Malaviya AN, Sharma A, Agarwal D, et al. Acute abdomen in SLE. Int J Rheum Dis. 2011; 14(1):98–104.

[50] Xu D, Yang H, Lai C-C, et al. Clinical analysis of systemic lupus erythematosus with gastrointestinal manifestations. Lupus 2010; 19(7):866–869.

Chapter 7

Physiotherapy Following Emergency Abdominal Surgery

Kate Sullivan, Julie Reeve, Ianthe Boden and Rebecca Lane

Additional information is available at the end of the chapter

http://dx.doi.org/10.5772/63969

Abstract

Physiotherapy following elective abdominal surgery has been well documented, but following emergency abdominal surgery, despite poorer outcomes and increased complication rates, physiotherapy interventions for this patient group remain largely uninvestigated. The most common complication following upper abdominal surgery is the development of a post-operative pulmonary complication (PPC). Risk factors for the development of PPCs include duration of anaesthesia, emergency upper abdominal surgery, current smoker status, respiratory comorbidities, obesity, increased age and multiple surgeries. Physiotherapy interventions aim to prevent or remediate PPCs and post-operative complications associated with the sequelae of immobility such as venothrombotic events and to facilitate recovery from surgery and a return to normal activities of daily living and function. Physiotherapy interventions after major surgery include early mobilisation and respiratory physiotherapy techniques. Respiratory therapies include deep breathing and coughing exercises, positive expiratory pressure devices, incentive spirometry and non-invasive ventilation. Early mobilisation has been demonstrated to be safe and efficacious following elective abdominal surgery and for patients who are critically ill. This chapter reviews the evidence in these populations and propose that, until further studies are available to direct care, this evidence is extrapolated to patients following emergency abdominal surgery. As abdominal surgery impacts on physical recovery and health-related quality of life, post-discharge rehabilitation programmes may improve long-term outcomes; however, rehabilitation following major cavity surgery is in its infancy. This chapter investigates post-operative rehabilitation research to date in this population in an attempt to determine the effectiveness of such programmes and make recommendations for future practice.

Keywords: physiotherapy, post-operative complications, emergency surgery, abdominal surgery, rehabilitation

1. Introduction

Recovery after abdominal surgery is multifaceted and requires input from a variety of health professionals. Recovery is not a concept that is well defined for healthcare professionals or for patients. Recovery has been previously described as a return to normality and wholeness through an energy requiring process and involves multiple domains, namely physical, physiological, psychological, social and economic [1, 2]. Physiotherapy aims to facilitate recovery from surgery by preventing or remediating post-operative complications and providing physical rehabilitation to assist a return to premorbid physical function, and whilst primarily focussing on physical rehabilitation, physiotherapy may impact on a number of the other domains. Rehabilitation commences, where possible, preoperatively and continues throughout the acute and sub-acute post-operative period and may extend beyond hospital discharge into community-based or ambulatory care to assist with a return to normal activities of daily living and function.

The effectiveness of physiotherapy to prevent complications and improve recovery for patients undergoing elective abdominal surgery has been well documented over the past 20 years [3]. However, despite data showing a higher incidence of complications and poorer physical recovery for patients undergoing emergency abdominal surgery [4, 5], the benefits of physiotherapy for this patient group are yet to be reported in detail.

This chapter will provide an overview of the common complications that occur following abdominal surgery including emergency surgery, specifically focussing on those that may be remediated by physiotherapy interventions. Evidence for physiotherapy interventions will be extrapolated based on both elective abdominal surgery studies and those combining elective and emergency surgical cohorts and recommendations for physiotherapy practice following emergency abdominal surgery will be presented.

2. Complications associated with emergency abdominal surgery

Physiotherapists have been involved in the routine provision of care to patients undergoing abdominal surgery since the 1950s [6, 7]. Post-operative complications are common following major upper abdominal surgery (UAS) with up to 50% of all patients having some type of complication following their surgery [8, 9]. Complications include post-operative pulmonary complications (PPCs), prolonged post-operative ileus, wound infection, haemorrhage and venothrombotic events [4]. Complications following emergency UAS are two to three times more common compared with similar elective procedures [4] with patients more susceptible to cardiopulmonary complications and sepsis [10]. These types of complications are shown to be the most frequent cause of early post-operative death and correspondingly the 30-day mortality rate is five times higher following emergency surgery compared with elective abdominal surgery [10].

2.1. Post-operative pulmonary complications

Post-operative pulmonary complications (PPCs) are described as '…a pulmonary abnormality that produces identifiable disease or dysfunction, that is clinically significant and adversely affects the clinical course' [11]. PPCs may include pneumonia, respiratory failure, atelectasis, sputum retention, pneumothorax, pleural effusion and pleural oedema [12] (see **Figure 1**).

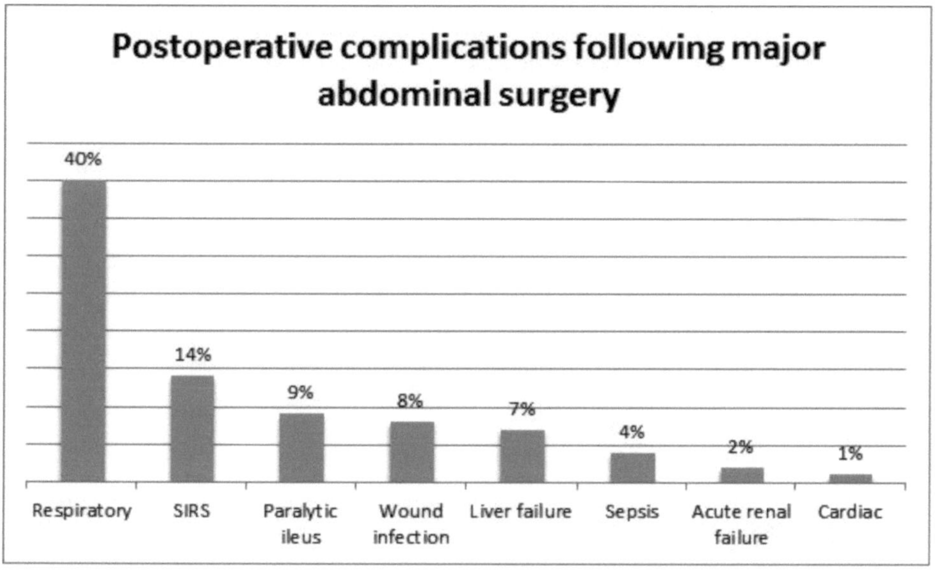

Figure 1. Post-operative complications following major elective abdominal surgery [12].

PPCs are a major cause of morbidity and mortality and the most common complication following elective UAS with a reported incidence of up to 40% [12]. Similar incidences of PPCs have been reported following emergency UAS [5, 10, 13, 14] although variability in the definition and diagnosis of PPC affects the reliability of this data [15]. Despite the true incidence being unclear, emergency surgery is seen as an independent risk factor for PPC across all surgery types [16].

PPCs have significant consequences for both the patient and healthcare services. Patients have poorer outcomes and a slower recovery if they develop a PPC following abdominal surgery. Hospital costs are doubled [17], length of stay is longer by a minimum of four days [18, 19], and mortality is higher [20, 21] in those patients who are diagnosed with a PPC following elective UAS. Considering the consequences of respiratory complications, much focus has been placed on their prevention. By identifying the factors that predispose to the development of

PPCs and the populations most at risk, prophylactic therapeutic interventions can be more appropriately targeted.

2.1.1. Risks factors associated with the development of PPCs

The pathophysiological effects of abdominal surgery on the respiratory system are well known. Atelectasis [22], alterations in mucociliary transport [23], respiratory muscle dysfunction and altered chest wall mechanics [5, 22], reduced lung volumes and decreased cough strength [22] are thought to contribute to an increased risk of PPC through the combined impact of general anaesthesia, post-operative pain and immobilisation, and handling of the viscera [22].

Factors most highly associated with the development of PPCs for patients undergoing elective abdominal surgery include duration of anaesthesia greater than 3 hours, upper gastrointestinal surgery, a current or recently ceased smoking history, estimated VO_2max below 19.37 ml/kg/min and respiratory co-morbidity [24]. Risk analysis from a recent study focussing on emergency upper and lower abdominal surgery identified age, abnormal body mass index, upper abdominal incision and multiple surgeries as predictors of PPC [5].

2.1.2. Identifying PPCs

Rates of PPC vary greatly depending on the diagnostic criteria used to define them, and such inconsistencies make identifying clinically significant PPCs, comparison of PPC rates and interpretation of research findings problematic. Additionally, not all clinically significant PPCs are amenable to physiotherapy interventions, for example, a pneumothorax. One diagnostic

Melbourne Group Score PPC diagnostic criteria

Diagnosis confirmed when 4 or more of the following are present in a 24 hr period:

CLINICAL FACTORS

- New abnormal breath sounds on auscultation different to preoperative assessment
- Production of yellow or green sputum different to preoperative assessmen
- Pulse oximetry oxygen saturation (SpO_2) <90% on room air on more than one consecutive postoperative day
- Raised maximum oral temperature >38°C on more than one consecutive postoperative day

DIAGNOSTIC FACTORS

- Chest radiograph report of collapse/consolidation
- An unexplained WCC greater than 11 x 10^9/L
- Presence of infection on sputum culture report

OTHER

- Physician's diagnosis of pneumonia, respiratory tract infection, undefined respiratory problem.
- Prescription of an antibiotic for a respiratory infection

Figure 2. The Melbourne Group Score PPC diagnostic criteria.

tool, the Melbourne Group Score (MGS), has recently been used to identify those PPCs considered potentially responsive to physiotherapy interventions, for example severe atelectasis and pneumonia. Whilst the measurement properties of the MGS have not yet been fully demonstrated, the tool has been shown to have excellent inter- and intrarater reliability and good clinical utility when compared to other similar diagnostic tools [25].

The MGS tool is an eight-item checklist, identifying patients as having a PPC if they are positive for four of the eight criteria in a 24-hour period (see **Figure 2**).

To date, the MGS has been used following abdominal [18, 26–28] and thoracic surgery [25, 29], and whilst further studies investigating its clinimetric properties are warranted, it currently remains the best tool for physiotherapists to determine the presence of a PPC amenable to their care.

2.2. Complications associated with prolonged immobility

Prolonged bed rest is associated with an increased risk of post-operative complications after surgery. Prolonged immobility has been shown to increase the risk of venous thromboembolism [30], result in loss of muscle bulk and strength [31], increase insulin resistance [32], reduce pulmonary function and tissue oxygenation and increase levels of hospital associated depression [33]. All of these complications increase patient length of hospital stay (LOS) and, in some cases such as venous thromboembolisation and decreased pulmonary function, can threaten life. More recently, literature has clearly demonstrated an increase in the risk of severe acute weakness syndromes such as intensive care unit-acquired weakness (ICUAW) in the context of sepsis and critical illness [34]. These weakness syndromes impact patients both during their acute recovery and following discharge, with some patients experiencing ongoing weakness and functional difficulties up to two years after their ICU discharge [34].

Delayed ambulation has also been associated with PPCs, with an observational cohort study finding patients were three times more likely to have a PPC diagnosis for each day they did not mobilise away from the bedside [27], although it is possible that the presence of a PPC caused the delay in ambulation rather than vice versa, as a majority of PPCs are diagnosed on the first post-operative day and before to the opportunity for early ambulation. Whilst no conclusive evidence has demonstrated that delayed ambulation increases the likelihood of a PPC, it does contribute to functional decline. A randomised controlled trial found that in patients following elective abdominal surgery where mobilisation was delayed by three days, more physiotherapy input was required, and length of hospital stay was increased by 4.4 days (95%CI 0.3–8.8) compared with those who ambulated on the first post-operative day [35].

2.3. Prolonged post-operative ileus

Post-operative ileus (POI) is a normal, transient impairment of bowel motility and is considered an inevitable consequence of abdominal surgery [36–38]. A clinically significant ileus, or prolonged ileus, is defined as lasting longer than three days [37, 39] and involves symptoms such as nausea and vomiting, inability to tolerate an oral diet, abdominal distension and delayed passage of flatus or stool [37, 38]. Prolonged ileus occurs in up to 25% of patients following major abdominal surgery, is associated with a higher risk of developing other post-operative complications and increases hospital length of stay [39]. Early ambulation is included as part of standard care guidelines and has been suggested to be influential on the timely resolution of ileus although there is currently little evidence for this [38]. Further studies are needed to test the hypothesis that early and frequent ambulation reduces ileus rates.

3. Physiotherapy following emergency abdominal surgery

To date, there have been limited data regarding physiotherapy interventions following emergency abdominal surgery. Physiotherapists caring for patients following emergency surgery can only base their interventions on evidence extrapolated from elective abdominal surgery and literature for critically ill patients.

Whilst preoperative education, inspiratory muscle training, and exercise training have been shown to significantly impact on PPCs in patients undergoing elective abdominal surgery [40–43], the nature of emergency surgery invariably renders this approach impossible in this patient group. Consequently, such patients are assumed at increased risk of post-operative complications.

3.1. Physiotherapy in the immediate post-operative period

Physiotherapists have been involved in the routine provision of care to patients undergoing abdominal surgery under the assumption that complications can be prevented by assisted early ambulation and respiratory physiotherapy techniques such as deep breathing and coughing (DB&C) exercises [44–46]. Whilst there is little evidence demonstrating effective physiotherapy techniques specifically for the emergency UAS population, there is good quality evidence to demonstrate that physiotherapy focusing on early rehabilitation in the immediate post-operative period is both safe and effective following elective UAS, and for patients with a critical illness (including following emergency surgery) in intensive care. As such, until further evidence becomes available, evidence from both the critical illness literature and the elective abdominal surgical literature should be applied to determine appropriate and effective interventions for these patients. Therapy usually comprises of early assisted mobilisation, respiratory physiotherapy, strength and conditioning rehabilitation and education.

3.1.1. Physiotherapy assessment

Physiotherapy assessment occurs in the context of the patient condition, the nature and type of the surgery, the ongoing medical plan, the patient's premorbid status and any comorbidities impacting upon post-operative rehabilitation. Level of alertness, ability to follow instructions and haemodynamic and respiratory stability will be carefully assessed before any therapeutic intervention is considered. Consensus guidelines for physiotherapy assessment and treatment have been recently published and, where higher quality evidence is absent, should be used as the primary resource for recommendations for physiotherapy practice [46].

3.1.2. Physiotherapy treatment

3.1.2.1. Early ambulation and rehabilitation

Early ambulation and rehabilitation have been extensively researched after both elective abdominal surgery and after critical illness. There is an increasingly compelling body of evidence that physical activity 1–2 times per day for up to 15–30 min is both safe and efficacious for critically ill patients [47]. Early mobilisation has been shown to decrease ICU and hospital length of stay, reduce the effect of ICUAW and improve quality of life [48]. Early mobilisation in the critically ill should be undertaken under highly controlled circumstances and such decisions are made according to individual patient status and haemodynamic stability. Evidence shows that adverse events occur in only a small number of patients (1–4%) [47, 49–52]. A recent systematic review reported no serious adverse medical consequences whilst mobilising critically ill patients in 14 of 15 trials [53].

Enhanced Recovery After Surgery (ERAS) protocols exist to inform peri-operative management of specific elective abdominal surgeries. Such protocols contain recommendations regarding, amongst other interventions, the importance of early ambulation after abdominal surgery, specifying the frequency and duration required to be undertaken. For example, for patients undergoing elective rectal or pelvic surgery the guidelines recommend they are nursed in an environment encouraging independence and mobilisation with two hours out of bed on the day of surgery and six hours out of bed each day thereafter [54]. A further example includes patients following elective pancreaticoduodenectomy and states such patients should be actively mobilised from the morning of the first post-operative day, with mobilisation targets to be met each day [55]. Regardless of specific protocols, there is general consensus that to counteract the deleterious effects of immobility following any abdominal surgery patients should be mobilised early and often [54–58].

3.1.2.2. Respiratory physiotherapy

Whilst DB&C exercises to clear secretions have previously been considered essential in physiotherapy programmes following abdominal surgery [46], there has been no convincing evidence showing them to be any more effective in reducing PPC incidence than providing frequent early intensive ambulation alone [59]. As a result, recent research has focussed on the effectiveness of providing early ambulation alone in preventing post-operative complications [46]. Following emergency UAS, some patients may be unable to ambulate due to, for example, haemodynamic instability or traumatic injury, and thus, the inclusion of DB&C should be considered to be of value after emergency UAS [46]. If sputum retention occurs post-operatively, DB&C can also be augmented using additional techniques such as positive expiratory pressure (PEP) therapies. Such devices have been purported to aid in improving lung volumes and secretion clearance although a systematic review concluded that PEP conveys no additional benefit over other respiratory techniques [60]. These findings were limited by the poor quality of studies and small samples sizes within the review. However, since this systematic review, a well-designed randomised controlled trial (RCT) has found that an oscillating PEP device reduced days of fever and LOS [61] following elective UAS and thoracic surgery.

Incentive spirometries (ISs) are respiratory devices, which aim to increase inspiratory volumes. Incentive spirometry has been researched extensively, but meta-analysis of the available data has found little benefit when administered prophylactically following elective surgery [62, 63]. The benefits of PEP and IS are currently unknown in emergency surgery populations; however, considering that emergency abdominal surgery patients are at high risk of PPC and that these devices are generally low cost, on the balance of risk versus benefit, such devices should be considered as a prophylactic respiratory physiotherapy treatment in patients considered high risk for the development of a PPC.

To date, the current research investigating the effectiveness of respiratory physiotherapy interventions in a population following emergency UAS is inconclusive due to limited low-quality research and poor sample sizes. In this high-risk population, it is possible that the benefit of a reduction in PPCs by the delivery of prophylactic low-cost, low-risk interventions may outweigh the high cost of PPCs to the healthcare system however further and better-quality research, including cost-benefit analyses, is required to determine this.

3.1.2.3. Non-invasive ventilation

Non-invasive ventilation (NIV) in the form of either continuous positive airway pressure (CPAP) or bi-level positive airway pressure (BiPAP) reverses the known reduction in functional residual capacity (FRC) following abdominal surgery. Mechanically driven air-flow (with or without additional oxygenation) is delivered during inspiration via a sealed facemask or nasal interface until a predetermined inspiratory positive airway pressure is obtained. On expiration, positive airway pressure is maintained with the use of a positive end expiratory pressure (PEEP) valve. This positive intrathoracic pressure throughout the breath cycle increases FRC, reverses atelectasis and improves gas exchange. NIV can be used either prophylactically aiming to prevent PPC, or as a therapy to address hypoxemia and respiratory failure.

Systematic reviews support the use of NIV to prevent respiratory complications following abdominal surgery despite methodological limitations of the clinical trials included. The majority of trials compared NIV to usual care of oxygen therapy alone and/or respiratory physiotherapy (DB&C ± incentive spirometry/PEP) in the post-operative period. These trials demonstrate NIV may reduce PPC risk by half, with a further significant sub-group effect specifically for the prevention of pneumonia [64, 65]. Systematic reviews and meta-analyses of NIV as a treatment for respiratory failure following abdominal surgery have not yet been performed due to the lack of clinical trials on this topic. However, a recent multicentre RCT has reported that NIV as a treatment for acute hypoxemic respiratory failure following abdominal surgery prevents tracheal intubation and reduces mortality when compared to using oxygen therapy alone [66].

Despite evidence supporting the use of NIV as an effective therapeutic intervention to prevent PPC, the uptake in hospitals is poor. Data from an observational study at a single large tertiary metropolitan hospital investigating PPC following high-risk abdominal surgery reported that NIV was utilised in just 3% of patients [13]. A reasonable question arises; if NIV has been shown to be superior to usual care in the prevention of PPC following abdominal surgery, why is it that this therapy is not widely provided as standard care? The answer to this question is likely to be multifactorial [67]. Clinical trials have not reported widely on the rates of negative effects of NIV. Potential risks and negative factors associated with the use of NIV are patient discomfort with the sealed interface leading to non-compliance, aspiration pneumonia secondary to emesis whilst wearing the mask, gastric gas insufflation, reduced venous return and cardiac filling, failure to provide consistent therapeutic pressure with air leaks around the interface occurring especially with the presence of nasogastric tubes, and the requirement for a dedicated skilled health professional to apply, titrate and to monitor the use of NIV making it problematic to manage outside the critical care environment. It may be that a combination of these negative factors prevents a hospital from providing this efficacious preventative therapy to all patients following abdominal surgery. Additionally, the paucity of cost-benefit and risk analysis evidence for NIV versus standard care may also be a factor. The hospital and patient costs of blanket NIV application may outweigh the benefit of preventing PPC, especially if the PPC incidence rate is low. Until detailed cost-benefit analysis and adverse event rates are reported in more detail, this remains unknown. It may not be necessary or cost-effective to treat all patients with prophylactic NIV. It may be more appropriate to stratify patients into high- and low-risk groups. Simple, low-cost prophylactic measures such as self-directed DB&C exercises, IS or PEP devices may be all that is required to prevent a PPC from occurring after low-risk abdominal surgery. Selective application of NIV to patients identified as being at high risk of developing a PPC may be more appropriate [68].

Other factors that need further investigation is the ideal frequency and duration of NIV therapy to prevent PPC, and, whether or not delivering high-flow humidified oxygen via specialised nasal prongs is as effective and/or more cost-effective as NIV in preventing PPC following abdominal surgery. Preliminary data have shown that high-flow nasal prongs (HFNP) are comparable to NIV in the treatment of hypoxemic respiratory failure yet with better patient compliance [69]. The use of HFNP following abdominal surgery to prevent PPC may be more a more feasible option compared with NIV and should be explored further.

Non-invasive ventilation is a proven prophylactic intervention in the reduction in PPC and pneumonia. Despite the evidence, application on a broad-scale is poor. On the balance of available evidence, prophylactic delivery of NIV should be targeted towards all patients at high risk of developing a PPC and this includes all patients having emergency open upper abdominal surgery.

3.1.2.4. Barriers to physiotherapy interventions

3.1.2.4.1. Cardiovascular and haemodynamic instability

In those undergoing emergency upper abdominal surgery, early mobilisation and other physiotherapy interventions may not be possible due to the increased likelihood of post-operative complications such as hypotension, post-operative bleeding and increased pain. It has been reported that following elective and emergency abdominal surgery, 52% of patients have some type of barrier to early ambulation with the most common being hypotension [13] although, where required respiratory therapies, such as DB&C, can all be applied in patients unable to mobilise unless contraindicated.

3.1.2.4.2. *Psychological preparedness*

In patients awaiting elective UAS, education and planning allows for some manner of psychological preparedness for surgery and what it entails. ERAS guidelines have recommendations regarding preoperative preparation of patients undergoing elective UAS with preoperative counselling recommended in all guidelines [54–58]. Emergency surgery leaves little or no time to prepare patients psychologically for the surgery or for the process of recovery after surgery. Post-operative education, detailing the rationale for respiratory care and early ambulation, is important to ensure patients are engaged in their own recovery and understand the necessity for complication prevention.

3.1.3. *Outcome measures*

The use of standardised outcome measures throughout the period of care provides a means to quantify change from baseline status and evaluate the efficacy of care. Emergency UAS dictates that premorbid status is often unknown and the impact of the surgery and subsequent rehabilitation on physical function may be unclear. Utilising standardised and repeatable outcome measures early in the post-operative period will provide a means by which changes in condition may be measured. These may include, but not be limited to respiratory, cardiovascular, musculoskeletal and neurological status. Studies investigating physiotherapy rehabilitation practices in acute surgical care commonly report LOS and post-operative complications as proxy outcome measures, but these measures have limitations when demonstrating the functional changes associated with physiotherapy interventions [70]. Outcome measures designed for the measurement of physical function in the acute care environment include, amongst others, the Physical Function ICU Test (PFIT) [71], the Acute Care Index of Function [70], Activity Measure for Post-Acute Care (AM-PAC) '6-Clicks' tool [72], the Modified Iowa Level of Assistance scale (mILOA) [73] and the Functional Independence Measure (FIM) [74, 75]. No single physical therapy functional outcome measure has yet been found to be valid and reliable specifically in patients following elective or emergency UAS. However, the PFIT and Acute Care Index of Function were developed for measuring mobility in patients with critical illness and the mILOA has been shown to be reliable, valid and responsive in assessing the mobility status of acute hospital inpatients [73] and their use could be extrapolated to the emergency surgery population. Determining tools with satisfactory psychometric and clinimetric properties in patients undergoing both elective and emergency abdominal surgery warrants further investigation. Embedding outcome measures should be a matter of routine in clinical practice and research and until a specific outcome measure for physical function is tested for the emergency UAS population, the use of well-tested outcome measures from other clinical populations is required.

3.1.4. Physiotherapy following discharge from hospital

Surgical and perioperative care should strive to improve both the quantity (life expectancy) and quality of life [76]. The development of even minor post-operative complications has been demonstrated to be a major determinant of hospital readmission, long-term adverse outcomes and death [77, 78]. Complications in the immediate post-operative period have been shown to be independent predictors of poorer recovery and poor Health Related Quality of Life (HRQoL) [79, 80] with delayed recovery and persistent disability following UAS demonstrated up to 6 months post-operatively [79]. Following major intestinal surgery in elderly patients, mortality, LOS, complication rate, discharge destination and discharge home with/without help were found to be significantly better in patients undergoing electively surgery compared with the same procedures performed as an emergency. Louis et al. [81] found 69% of patients were discharged directly home after elective procedures compared with only 6.5% if the same procedure was performed as an emergency. Less than half of older adults admitted to hospital for any cause return to their premorbid function within 1 year [82]. Despite these studies, little work has been done to investigate what ongoing rehabilitation support patients require or is available following emergency abdominal surgery. Indeed, it has been argued that after emergency surgery, future studies should reconsider their focus and consider utilising long-term functional outcomes alongside more traditional outcomes such as in-hospital or 30-day mortality and morbidity [81]. It is conceivable that following abdominal surgery post-operative exercise rehabilitation programmes (both in the inpatient and outpatient environment) might hasten recovery, alter discharge destination and improve long-term outcomes.

Whilst caution is warranted in extrapolating data from Louis et al. [81] to patients following emergency abdominal surgery, the feasibility of inpatient rehabilitation programmes has been determined in recent studies for patients recovering from critical illness [83, 84]. In this phase of recovery, the aim of improving physical function to promote safe and timely hospital discharge is similar across populations. Beyond hospital discharge, to date only a small number of studies exist which investigate the effect of post-discharge rehabilitation programmes and none of these are solely in patients undergoing abdominal surgery [85–89]. Recently, a Cochrane systematic review [90] has examined the effect of physical rehabilitation on HRQoL and physical recovery following critical illness and ICU stay. The review included six clinical trials (483 adult ICU participants) that compared an exercise intervention after ICU discharge with any other intervention or a control/usual care programme in adult survivors of critical illness. The overall quality of the evidence precluded meta-analysis. The exercise-based interventions were delivered as inpatient programmes in two studies, as both inpatient and outpatients in one study and as outpatients in three studies. Whilst the duration of the intervention varied according to length of hospital stay following ICU discharge, it was generally for a period of 12 weeks. Outcome measures were functional exercise capacity and HRQoL but these varied in both their measurement and the tool used for measurement. Overall, the quality of the evidence was low and study findings were inconsistent; some studies reported improvements in functional exercise capacity and others not. The review found no effect on HRQoL.

Given the absence of evidence investigating the effect of rehabilitation programmes on patients having undergone elective or emergency abdominal surgery, and the limitations in the evidence in a population following critical illness, further investigation of the value of post-discharge physical rehabilitation programmes is warranted.

4. Recommendations for physiotherapy practice in patients following emergency abdominal surgery

Patient education regarding the necessity for physiotherapy interventions should be implemented post-operatively as soon as feasible to ensure patients are engaged in their own recovery and understand complication prevention strategies such as respiratory physiotherapy and early mobilisation.

Mobilisation should be commenced as soon as possible to prevent complications associated with prolonged immobility.

Evidence for the prophylactic use of DB&C exercises, PEP or IS in patients following emergency abdominal surgery is generally of low quality and under-powered. Until further evidence is available to guide best practice, DB&C exercises should be instituted where ambulation is delayed in high-risk patients. Incentive spirometry and PEP devices can be provided prophylactically on a case-by-case basis where individual hospitals decide that the benefit of reducing PPC outweighs the cost of this service provision.

There is evidence to suggest prophylactic NIV is effective in preventing PPCs following abdominal surgery. The cost-effectiveness associated with providing prophylactic NIV to all patients undergoing abdominal surgery has not been established, and thus, it is recommended that the use of post-operative NIV is restricted to those at high risk of developing a PPC.

For audit, research and clinical purposes, the Melbourne Group Score should be used to diagnose PPCs that are amenable to physiotherapy intervention.

Evidence for post-discharge rehabilitation is lacking. In the absence of evidence, we recommend assessment of functional ability on discharge from hospital to highlight patients who may require ongoing rehabilitation.

5. Conclusion

Complications following emergency abdominal surgery include PPCs and the sequelae of prolonged immobility. Physiotherapy aims to remediate these problems, but to date, the effectiveness of these interventions in patients following emergency abdominal surgery has been poorly investigated. Due to paucity of published physiotherapy outcome data in this patient group, we have drawn on evidence from patients with critical illness or undergoing elective abdominal surgery to enable us to make recommendations for practice; however, we recognise the limitations with adopting this approach. The chapter has attempted to highlight the areas for further research to help determine the effectiveness of physiotherapy interventions in this high-risk patient population.

Author details

Kate Sullivan[1,2,3], Julie Reeve[4], Ianthe Boden[2,3,5*] and Rebecca Lane[1]

*Address all correspondence to: ianthe.boden@ths.tas.gov.au

1 School of Primary Health Care, Faculty of Nursing, Medicine and Health Science, Monash University, Frankston, Victoria, Australia

2 Physiotherapy Department, Launceston General Hospital, Launceston, Tasmania, Australia

3 Clifford Craig Medical Research Trust, Launceston General Hospital, Launceston, Tasmania, Australia

4 School of Rehabilitation and Occupation Studies, Faculty of Health and Environmental Sciences, Auckland University of Technology, Auckland, New Zealand

5 Department of Physiotherapy, Melbourne School of Health Sciences, The University of Melbourne, Parkville, Victoria, Australia

References

[1] Allvin R, Berg K, Idvall E, Nilsson U. Postoperative recovery: a concept analysis. Journal of Advanced Nursing. 2007;57(5):552–8.

[2] Lee L, Tran T, Mayo NE, Carli F, Feldman LS. What does it really mean to "recover" from an operation? Surgery. 2014;155(2):211–6.

[3] Reeve J, Boden I. The physiotherapy management of patients undergoing abdominal surgery. New Zealand Journal of Physiotherapy. 2016;42(1):33–49.

[4] Sørensen LT, Malaki A, Wille-Jørgensen P, Kallehave F, Kjærgaard J, Hemmingsen U, et al. Risk factors for mortality and postoperative complications after gastrointestinal surgery. Journal of Gastrointestinal Surgery. 2007;11(7):903–10.

[5] Serejo LGG, da Silva-Júnior FP, Bastos JPC, de Bruin GS, Mota RMS, de Bruin PFC. Risk factors for pulmonary complications after emergency abdominal surgery. Respiratory Medicine. 2007;101(4):808–13.

[6] Cash J. Physiotherapy in Some Surgical Conditions. London: Faber and Faber; 1955. p. 105–44.

[7] Innocenti D. An overview of the development of breathing exercises into the specialty of physiotherapy for heart and lung conditions. Physiotherapy. 1996;82(12):681–93.

[8] Aahlin E, Tranø G, Johns N, Horn A, Søreide J, Fearon K, et al. Risk factors, complications and survival after upper abdominal surgery: a prospective cohort study. BMC Surgery. 2015;15(1):83.

[9] Hamel MB, Henderson WG, Khuri SF, Daley J. Surgical outcomes for patients aged 80 and older: morbidity and mortality from major noncardiac surgery. Journal of the American Geriatrics Society. 2005;53(3):424–9.

[10] Vester-Andersen M, Waldau T, Wetterslev J, Møller MH, Rosenberg J, Jørgensen LN, et al. Randomized multicentre feasibility trial of intermediate care versus standard ward care after emergency abdominal surgery (InCare trial). British Journal of Surgery. 2015;102(6):619–29. doi:10.1002/bjs.9749.

[11] O'Donohue Jr W. Postoperative pulmonary complications. When are preventive and therapeutic measures necessary? Postgraduate Medicine. 1992;91(3):167–70.

[12] PROVHILO group. High versus low positive end-expiratory pressure during general anaesthesia for open abdominal surgery (PROVHILO trial): a multicentre randomised controlled trial. Lancet. 2014;384(9942):495–503. doi: 10.1016/S0140-6736(14)60416-5.

[13] Haines KJ, Skinner EH, Berney S, Austin Health PSI. Association of postoperative pulmonary complications with delayed mobilisation following major abdominal surgery: an observational cohort study. Physiotherapy. 2013;99(2):119–25. doi:10.1016/j.physio.2012.05.013.

[14] Wilson I, Barrett MP, Sinha A, Chan S. Predictors of in-hospital mortality amongst octogenarians undergoing emergency general surgery: a retrospective cohort study. International Journal of Surgery. 2014;12(11):1157–61.

[15] Smetana GW. Preoperative pulmonary assessment of the older adult. Clinics in Geriatric Medicine. 2003;19(1):35–55.

[16] Canet J, Gallart L, Gomar C, Paluzie G, Valles J, Castillo J, et al. Prediction of postoperative pulmonary complications in a population-based surgical cohort. Anesthesiology. 2010;113(6):1338–50.

[17] Lång M, Niskanen M, Miettinen P, Alhava E, Takala J. Outcome and resource utilization in gastroenterological surgery. British Journal of Surgery. 2001;88(7):1006–14.

[18] Scholes RL, Browning L, Sztendur EM, Denehy L. Duration of anaesthesia, type of surgery, respiratory co-morbidity, predicted VO max and smoking predict postoperative pulmonary complications after upper abdominal surgery: an observational study. Australian Journal of Physiotherapy. 2009;55(3):191–8.

[19] Helgstrand F, Rosenberg J, Kehlet H, Bisgaard T. Nationwide analysis of prolonged hospital stay and readmission after elective ventral hernia repair. Danish Medical Bulletin. 2011;58(10):A4322.

[20] Arenal JJ, Bengoechea-Beeby M. Mortality associated with emergency abdominal surgery in the elderly. Canadian Journal of Surgery. 2003;46(2):111.

[21] Martínez-Serrano MÁ, Pereira JA, Sancho JJ, López-Cano M, Bombuy E, Hidalgo J. Risk of death after emergency repair of abdominal wall hernias. Still waiting for improvement. Langenbeck's Archives of Surgery. 2010;395(5):551–6.

[22] Warner DO. Preventing postoperative pulmonary complications the role of the anesthesiologist. The Journal of the American Society of Anesthesiologists. 2000;92(5): 1467–72.

[23] Gamsu G, Singer MM, Vincent HH, Berry S, Nadel JA. Postoperative Impairment of Mucous Transport in the Lung 1–4. American Review of Respiratory Disease. 1976;114(4):673–9.

[24] Scholes R, Browning L, Sztendur E, Denehy L. Duration of anaesthesia, type of surgery, respiratory co-morbidity, predicted VO2max and smoking predict postoperative pulmonary complications after upper abdominal surgery: an observational study. Australian Journal of Physiotherapy. 2009;55(3):191–8.

[25] Agostini P, Naidu B, Cieslik H, Rathinam S, Bishay E, Kalkat M, et al. Comparison of recognition tools for postoperative pulmonary complications following thoracotomy. Physiotherapy. 2011;97(4):278–83.

[26] Browning L, Denehy L, Scholes RL. The quantity of early upright mobilisation performed following upper abdominal surgery is low: an observational study. Australian Journal of Physiotherapy. 2007;53(1):47–52.

[27] Haines KJ, Skinner EH, Berney S. Association of postoperative pulmonary complications with delayed mobilisation following major abdominal surgery: an observational cohort study. Physiotherapy. 2013;99(2):119–25. doi:10.1016/j.physio.2012.05.013.

[28] Parry S, Denehy L, Berney S, Browning L. Clinical application of the Melbourne risk prediction tool in a high-risk upper abdominal surgical population: an observational cohort study. Physiotherapy. 2014;100(1):47–53.

[29] Reeve JC, Nicol K, Stiller K, McPherson KM, Birch P, Gordon IR, et al. Does physiotherapy reduce the incidence of postoperative pulmonary complications following pulmonary resection via open thoracotomy? A preliminary randomised single-blind clinical trial. European Journal of Cardio-Thoracic Surgery. 2010;37(5):1158–66.

[30] Cassidy MR, Rosenkranz P, McAneny D. Reducing postoperative venous thromboembolism complications with a standardized risk-stratified prophylaxis protocol and mobilization program. Journal of the American College of Surgeons. 2014;218(6): 1095–104.

[31] Ringholm S, Biensø RS, Kiilerich K, Guadalupe-Grau A, Aachmann-Andersen NJ, Saltin B, et al. Bed rest reduces metabolic protein content and abolishes exercise-induced mRNA responses in human skeletal muscle. American Journal of Physiology-Endocrinology and Metabolism. 2011;301(4):E649–E58.

[32] Biensø RS, Ringholm S, Kiilerich K, Aachmann-Andersen N-J, Krogh-Madsen R, Guerra B, et al. GLUT4 and glycogen synthase are key players in bed rest-induced insulin resistance. Diabetes. 2012;61(5):1090–9.

[33] Allen C, Glasziou P, Mar CD. Bed rest: a potentially harmful treatment needing more careful evaluation. The Lancet. 1999;354(9186):1229–33.

[34] Hermans G, Van den Berghe G. Clinical review: intensive care unit acquired weakness. Critical Care. 2015;19(1):1–9.

[35] Silva Y, Li S, Rickard M. Does the addition of deep breathing exercises to physiotherapy-directed early mobilisation alter patient outcomes following high-risk open upper abdominal surgery? Physiotherapy. 2013;99(3):187–93.

[36] Artinyan A, Nunoo-Mensah JW, Balasubramaniam S, Gauderman J, Essani R, Gonzalez-Ruiz C, et al. Prolonged postoperative ileus-definition, risk factors, and predictors after surgery. World Journal of Surgery. 2008;32(7):1495–500. doi:10.1007/s00268-008-9491-2.

[37] Millan M, Biondo S, Fraccalvieri D, Frago R, Golda T, Kreisler E. Risk factors for prolonged postoperative ileus after colorectal cancer surgery. World Journal of Surgery. 2012;36(1):179–85. doi:10.1007/s00268-011-1339-5.

[38] Vather R, Trivedi S, Bissett I. Defining postoperative ileus: results of a systematic review and global survey. Journal of Gastrointestinal Surgery: Official Journal of the Society for Surgery of the Alimentary Tract. 2013;17(5):962–72. doi:10.1007/s11605-013-2148-y.

[39] Vather R, Bissett I. Management of prolonged post-operative ileus: evidence-based recommendations. ANZ Journal of Surgery. 2013;83(5):319–24. doi:10.1111/ans.12102.

[40] Fagevik Olsén M, Hahn I, Nordgren S, Lonroth H, Lundholm K. Randomized controlled trial of prophylactic chest physiotherapy in major abdominal surgery. British Journal of Surgery. 1997;84(11):1535–8.

[41] Samnani SS, Umer MF, Mehdi SH, Farid FN. Impact of preoperative counselling on early postoperative mobilization and its role in smooth recovery. International Scholarly Research Notices. 2014:1–4.

[42] Mans CM, Reeve JC, Elkins MR. Postoperative outcomes following preoperative inspiratory muscle training in patients undergoing cardiothoracic or upper abdominal surgery: a systematic review and meta analysis. Clinical Rehabilitation. 2014. doi: 10.1177/0269215514545350.

[43] Pouwels S, Stokmans RA, Willigendael EM, Nienhuijs SW, Rosman C, van Ramshorst B, et al. Preoperative exercise therapy for elective major abdominal surgery: a system-

atic review. International Journal of Surgery. 2014;12(2):134–40. doi:10.1016/j.ijsu.2013.11.018.

[44] Makhabah DN, Martino F, Ambrosino N. Peri-operative physiotherapy. Multidisciplinary Respiratory Medicine. 2013;8(1):4.

[45] Smetana GW. Postoperative pulmonary complications: an update on risk assessment and reduction. Cleveland Clinic Journal of Medicine. 2009;76(Suppl 4):S60–S5.

[46] Hanekom S, Brooks D, Denehy L, Fagevik-Olsen M, Hardcastle T, Manie S, et al. Reaching consensus on the physiotherapeutic management of patients following upper abdominal surgery: a pragmatic approach to interpret equivocal evidence. BMC Medical Informatics and Decision Making. 2012;6:12.

[47] Perme C, Chandrashekar R. Early mobility and walking program for patients in intensive care units: creating a standard of care. American Journal of Critical Care. 2009;18(3):212–21.

[48] Kress JP. Clinical trials of early mobilization of critically ill patients. Critical Care Medicine. 2009;37(10):S442–S7.

[49] Mendez-Tellez PA, Nusr R, Feldman D, Needham DM. Early physical rehabilitation in the ICU: a review for the neurohospitalist. The Neurohospitalist. 2012;2(3):96–105.

[50] Thomas AJ. Physiotherapy led early rehabilitation of the patient with critical illness. Physical Therapy Reviews. 2011;16(1):46–57.

[51] Truong AD, Fan E, Brower RG, Needham DM. Bench-to-bedside review: mobilizing patients in the intensive care unit–from pathophysiology to clinical trials. Critical Care. 2009;13(4):216.

[52] Castro-Avila AC, Serón P, Fan E, Gaete M, Mickan S. Effect of early rehabilitation during intensive care unit stay on functional status: systematic review and meta-analysis. PloS One. 2015;10(7).

[53] Adler J, Malone D. Early mobilization in the intensive care unit: a systematic review. Cardiopulmonary Physical Therapy Journal. 2012;23(1):5.

[54] Nygren J, Thacker J, Carli F, Fearon K, Norderval S, Lobo D, et al. Guidelines for perioperative care in elective rectal/pelvic surgery: Enhanced Recovery After Surgery (ERAS®) Society recommendations. Clinical Nutrition. 2012;31(6):801–16.

[55] Lassen K, Coolsen MM, Slim K, Carli F, de Aguilar-Nascimento JE, Schäfer M, et al. Guidelines for perioperative care for pancreaticoduodenectomy: Enhanced Recovery After Surgery (ERAS®) Society recommendations. Clinical Nutrition. 2012;31(6):817–30.

[56] Cerantola Y, Valerio M, Persson B, Jichlinski P, Ljungqvist O, Hubner M, et al. Guidelines for perioperative care after radical cystectomy for bladder cancer: Enhanced

Recovery After Surgery (ERAS®) society recommendations. Clinical Nutrition. 2013;32(6):879–87.

[57] Gustafsson U, Scott M, Schwenk W, Demartines N, Roulin D, Francis N, et al. Guidelines for perioperative care in elective colonic surgery: Enhanced Recovery After Surgery (ERAS®) Society recommendations. Clinical Nutrition. 2012;31(6):783–800.

[58] Mortensen K, Nilsson M, Slim K, Schäfer M, Mariette C, Braga M, et al. Consensus guidelines for enhanced recovery after gastrectomy. British Journal of Surgery. 2014;101(10):1209–29.

[59] Mackay M, Ellis E, Johnston C. Randomised clinical trial of physiotherapy after open abdominal surgery in high risk patients. Australian Journal of Physiotherapy. 2005;51(3):151–9.

[60] Orman J, Westerdahl E. Chest physiotherapy with positive expiratory pressure breathing after abdominal and thoracic surgery: a systematic review (structured abstract). Acta Anaesthesiologica Scandinavica. 2010.

[61] Zhang XY, Wang Q, Zhang S, Tan W, Wang Z, Li J. The use of a modified, oscillating positive expiratory pressure device reduced fever and length of hospital stay in patients after thoracic and upper abdominal surgery: a randomised trial. Journal of Physiotherapy. 2015;61(1):16–20. doi:10.1016/j.jphys.2014.11.013.

[62] Freitas Eliane RFS, Soares Bernardo GO, Cardoso Jefferson R, Atallah Álvaro N. Incentive spirometry for preventing pulmonary complications after coronary artery bypass graft. Cochrane Database of Systematic Reviews. 2012. doi: 10.1002/14651858.CD004466.pub3.

[63] do Nascimento Junior P, Módolo Norma SP, Andrade S, Guimarães Michele MF, Braz Leandro G, El Dib R. Incentive spirometry for prevention of postoperative pulmonary complications in upper abdominal surgery. Cochrane Database of Systematic Reviews. 2014. doi:10.1002/14651858.CD006058.pub3.

[64] Ireland CJ, Chapman TM, Mathew SF, Herbison GP, Zacharias M. Continuous positive airway pressure (CPAP) during the postoperative period for prevention of postoperative morbidity and mortality following major abdominal surgery. Cochrane Database of Systematic Reviews. 2014;8.

[65] Ferreyra GP, Baussano I, Squadrone V, Richiardi L, Marchiaro G, Del Sorbo L, et al. Continuous positive airway pressure for treatment of respiratory complications after abdominal surgery: a systematic review and meta-analysis. Annals of Surgery. 2008;247(4):617–26.

[66] Jaber S, Lescot T, Futier E, Paugam-Burtz C, Seguin P, Ferrandiere M, et al. Effect of noninvasive ventilation on tracheal reintubation among patients with hypoxemic respiratory failure following abdominal surgery: a randomized clinical trial. JAMA. 2016;315(13):1345–53.

[67] Harvey G, Kitson A. Translating evidence into healthcare policy and practice: single versus multi-faceted implementation strategies—is there a simple answer to a complex question? International Journal of Health Policy and Management. 2015;4(3):123.

[68] Fiore JF, Chiavegato LD, Paisani DM, Colucci DB. Utilization of positive-pressure devices for breathing exercises in the hospital setting: a regional survey in Sao Paulo, Brazil. Respiratory Care. 2010;55(6):719–24.

[69] Frat J-P, Thille AW, Mercat A, Girault C, Ragot S, Perbet S, et al. High-flow oxygen through nasal cannula in acute hypoxemic respiratory failure. New England Journal of Medicine. 2015;372(23):2185–96.

[70] Scherer SA, Hammerich AS. Outcomes in cardiopulmonary physical therapy: acute care index of function. Cardiopulmonary Physical Therapy Journal. 2008;19(3):94–7.

[71] Berney S, Skinner E, Denehy L, Warrillow S. Development of a physical function outcome measure (PFIT) and a pilot exercise training protocol for use in intensive care. Critical Care and Resuscitation. 2009;11(2):110.

[72] Jette DU, Stilphen M, Ranganathan VK, Passek SD, Frost FS, Jette AM. Validity of the AM-PAC "6-Clicks" inpatient daily activity and basic mobility short forms. Physical Therapy. 2014;94(3):379–91.

[73] Kimmel LA, Elliott JE, Sayer JM, Holland AE. Assessing the reliability and validity of a physical therapy functional measurement tool—the modified iowa level of assistance scale—in acute hospital inpatients. Physical Therapy. 2015.

[74] Granger CV, Hamilton BB, Keith RA, Zielezny M, Sherwin FS. Advances in functional assessment for medical rehabilitation. Topics in Geriatric Rehabilitation. 1986;1(3):59–74.

[75] Bohannon RW, Leary KM. Standing balance and function over the course of acute rehabilitation. Archives of Physical Medicine and Rehabilitation. 1995;76(11):994–6.

[76] Peden C, Grocott M. National research strategies: what outcomes are important in perioperative elderly care? Anaesthesia. 2014;69(s1):61–9.

[77] Moonesinghe S, Harris S, Mythen M, Rowan K, Haddad F, Emberton M, et al. Survival after postoperative morbidity: a longitudinal observational cohort study. British Journal of Anaesthesia. 2014;113(6):977–84.

[78] Khuri SF, Henderson WG, DePalma RG, Mosca C, Healey NA, Kumbhani DJ. Determinants of long-term survival after major surgery and the adverse effect of postoperative complications. Annals of Surgery. 2005;242(3):326–43.

[79] Lawrence VA, Hazuda HP, Cornell JE, Pederson T, Bradshaw PT, Mulrow CD, et al. Functional independence after major abdominal surgery in the elderly. Journal of the American College of Surgeons. 2004;199(5):762–72.

[80] Davies SJ, Francis J, Dilley J, Wilson RJT, Howell SJ, Allgar V. Measuring outcomes after major abdominal surgery during hospitalization: reliability and validity of the Postoperative Morbidity Survey. Perioperative Medicine. 2013;2(1):1.

[81] Louis DJ, Hsu A, Brand MI, Saclarides TJ. Morbidity and mortality in octogenarians and older undergoing major intestinal surgery. Diseases of the Colon & Rectum. 2009;52(1):59–63.

[82] Covinsky KE, Pierluissi E, Johnston CB. Hospitalization-associated disability:"She was probably able to ambulate, but I'm not sure". JAMA. 2011;306(16):1782–93.

[83] Salisbury L, Merriweather J, Walsh T. The development and feasibility of a ward-based physiotherapy and nutritional rehabilitation package for people experiencing critical illness. Clinical Rehabilitation. 2010;24(6):489–500.

[84] Denehy L, Berney S, Skinner E, Edbrooke L, Haines K, Warrillow S, et al. Evaluation of exercise rehabilitation for survivors of intensive care: an assessor blinded randomised controlled trial. American Journal of Respiratory and Critical Care Medicine. 2011;183:A2642.

[85] Connolly B, Denehy L, Brett S, Elliott D, Hart N. Exercise rehabilitation following hospital discharge in survivors of critical illness: an integrative review. Critical Care. 2012;16(3):226.

[86] Connolly B, Thompson A, Douiri A, Moxham J, Hart N. Exercise-based rehabilitation after hospital discharge for survivors of critical illness with intensive care unit–acquired weakness: a pilot feasibility trial. Journal of Critical Care. 2015;30(3):589–98.

[87] Elliott D, McKinley S, Alison J, Aitken LM, King M, Leslie GD, et al. Health-related quality of life and physical recovery after a critical illness: a multi-centre randomised controlled trial of a home-based physical rehabilitation program. Critical Care. 2011;15(3):R142.

[88] Jones C, Skirrow P, Griffiths RD, Humphris GH, Ingleby S, Eddleston J, et al. Rehabilitation after critical illness: a randomized, controlled trial. Critical Care Medicine. 2003;31(10):2456–61.

[89] Denehy L, Skinner EH, Edbrooke L, Haines K, Warrillow S, Hawthorne G, et al. Exercise rehabilitation for patients with critical illness: a randomized controlled trial with 12 months of follow-up. Critical Care. 2013;17(4):R156.

[90] Connolly B, Salisbury L, O'Neill B, Geneen L, Douiri A, Grocott M, et al. Exercise rehabilitation following intensive care unit discharge for recovery from critical illness. Cochrane Database of Systematic Reviews. 2015;6.

Section 2

Abdominal Trauma

Chapter 8

Traumatic Bile Duct Injuries

Michele Molinari

Additional information is available at the end of the chapter

http://dx.doi.org/10.5772/64535

Abstract

The vast majority of bile duct injuries is iatrogenic and occurs during abdominal surgeries or other interventions such as endoscopic or percutaneous cannulation of the biliary tree. Accidental traumas are responsible only for 1–5% of the total number of biliary injuries. The diagnosis of non-iatrogenic traumatic bile duct injuries is challenging as current cross-sectional imaging tests are not very specific. Therefore, most of the patients are diagnosed when they undergo early explorative laparotomy or when they develop late complications. Among all patients who experience traumatic bile duct injuries, 80–90% are victims of penetrating traumas from stab or gunshot wounds. On the other hand, bile duct lesions due to blunt traumas are predominantly caused by traffic accidents (compression by safety belt or airbag), falls, kicks, or work accidents. Iatrogenic bile duct injuries have been extensively covered in many other papers. In this chapter, we will focus our attention only on traumatic bile duct injuries.

Keywords: bile duct injuries, penetrating trauma, blunt trauma, endoscopic retrograde cholangiography, cholecystectomy, cholecystorrhaphy, biliary-enteric anastomosis, biloma, hemobilia

1. Introduction

Most of the bile duct injuries from traumas are associated with damage to the liver and present with a spectrum of conditions ranging from full transections or partial lacerations, to simple contusions and wall hematomas [1–12]. Eighty-five percent of patients diagnosed with extrahepatic biliary traumas suffer injuries of the gallbladder, whereas involvement of the main bile duct alone occurs only in 15% of the cases. In patients with injuries of the extrahepatic bile duct, the most frequent location is in the proximity of the hepatic hilum or within the head of the pancreas. Theories to explain this phenomenon are several. The most convincing is that blunt forces to the abdomen push the liver upward stretching the hepatoduodenal ligament to the point of disruption at the bile duct bifurcation. Moreover, in the proximity to the sphincter of Oddi there is already a physiologic elevation of the intraluminal pressure that is suddenly increased by the traumatic event causing disruption of the bile duct wall in this area. In patients affected by blunt trauma, the portal vein and hepatic artery are not usually injured because these structures are longer and more elastic than the main bile duct. Also, when patients suffer damage to vascular structures of the hepatoduodenal ligament, most of the times they do not survive the accident and are pronounced dead before arrival to the emergency department [1, 13–24].

2. Clinical presentation

The clinical presentation of patients with traumatic bile duct injuries has changed over the last few decades due to the different management of patients with blunt abdominal traumas. Currently, patients with a blunt trauma and who are hemodynamically stable or without signs of peritonitis are managed nonoperatively regardless of the severity and mechanism of their liver injuries [25, 26]. On the other hand, hemodynamically unstable patients or patients with peritoneal signs require an exploratory laparotomy. The primary goal during trauma laparotomies is to stop the hemorrhage and to prevent uncontrolled contamination of the peritoneal cavity by repairing defects of hollow viscera. Trauma laparotomies in these settings are referred as "damage controlled surgeries" (DCS) where the main goal is to control life-threatening conditions while more definitive treatments are necessary after patients are adequately resuscitated [27, 28].

3. Diagnosis of bile duct injuries

Injuries to the extrahepatic bile ducts are particularly rare and make up no more than 30% of biliary injuries, the vast majority being due to penetrating trauma [29–31]. There are three main diagnostic patterns of traumatic bile duct injuries. The first one is immediate identification during DCS. Patients with immediate diagnosis represent a challenging group as they require complex surgical interventions because they often have multiple other injuries.

The second one is diagnosis within the first week and includes 50% of patients with blunt traumas who present with hemodynamic stability and absence of peritoneal signs at the time of presentation in the emergency room. In these cases, cross-sectional imaging studies often show the presence of free intra-abdominal fluid. Radiologically, it is quite difficult to distinguish between blood and other types of fluids. Therefore, when indicated percutaneous drainage or peritoneal lavage is helpful to characterize the nature of the abdominal free fluid. The presence of elevated concentrations of amylase and bilirubin in the aspirate confirms the occurrence of a bile duct injury or intestinal perforation that will require surgical intervention. Other diagnostic modalities that can help in the differential diagnosis are hydroxy iminodi-

http://dx.doi.org/10.5772/64535

acetic acid (HIDA) scan, magnetic resonance cholangiography (MRCP), and endoscopic retrograde cholangiography (ERCP). Finally, a relatively small proportion of patients presents with late complications, often several months or years after their original trauma. These patients usually develop biliary strictures conditioning dilation of the proximal biliary tree with recurrent episodes of cholangitis or obstructive jaundice. In recent years, because of the growing adoption of nonsurgical approaches to the initial treatment of abdominal traumas, this group of patients has increased significantly.

4. Clinical definition of minor or major bile duct injuries

Minor bile duct leaks are defined as drainage of less than 400 ml of bile per day for a period shorter than 14 days. On the other hand, a major bile duct leak occurs when there is more than 400 ml of bilious drainage per day or more than 50 ml of bilious drainage each day for more than 14 days [32].

5. Anatomical classification and severity of bile duct injuries

Traumatic bile duct injuries can be classified in intrahepatic and extrahepatic. This classification not only identifies the anatomical location of the injuries, but also helps directing diagnostic modalities and treatment interventions.

5.1. Intrahepatic injuries

Intrahepatic biliary duct injuries are subcategorized into two groups according to where the injury occurs in the biliary tree. The first group includes central biliary injuries and the second group includes peripheral bile duct injuries. Central intrahepatic biliary injuries are those where the injury falls within 5 cm from the hepatic duct bifurcation. Peripheral biliary injuries

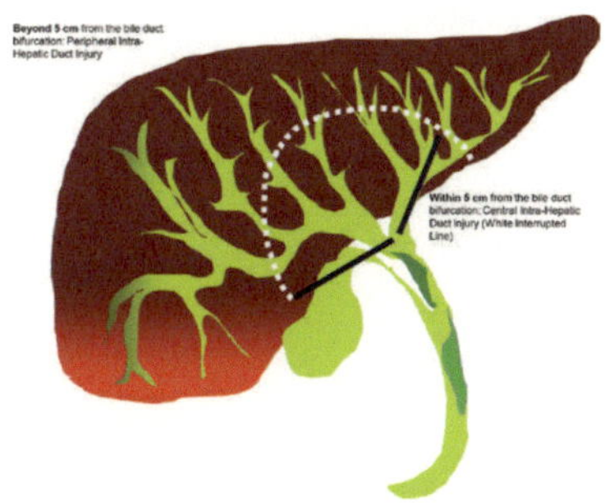

Figure 1. Schematic representation of the anatomical classification of intrahepatic biliary duct injuries. Central intrahepatic biliary duct injuries occur when the trauma affects biliary ducts within 5 cm from the biliary duct bifurcation. Peripheral intrahepatic bile duct injuries occur when the trauma affects hepatic parenchyma that is more than 5 cm distant from the bile duct bifurcation.

are those within the hepatic parenchyma affecting bile ducts that is more than 5 cm distant from the hepatic duct confluence (**Figure 1**) [33]. Since most of the intrahepatic bile duct injuries are associated with hepatic parenchyma damage, classification of this type of biliary injuries is often based on the liver injury scale as proposed by Moore et al. [34, 35] and summarized in **Table 1**.

Grade	Injury	ICD
I. Hematoma	Nonexpanding, subcapsular hematoma occupying less than 10% of surface area	846.01
I. Laceration	Nonbleeding, less than 1 cm deep capsular tear	864.11
II. Hematoma	Nonexpanding, subcapsular hematoma occupying 10–50% of surface area	864.01
	Nonexpanding intraparenchymal hematoma less than 2 cm in diameter	864.11
II. Laceration	Active bleeding, 1–3 cm deep capsular tear measuring less than 10 in length	864.03
III. Hematoma	Subcapsular hematoma more than 50% of surface area or expanding	864.04
	Ruptured subcapsular hematoma with active bleeding	
	Intraparenchymal hematoma larger than 2 cm or expanding	
III. Laceration	Deeper than 3 cm	864.04
IV. Hematoma	Ruptured intraparenchymal hematoma with active bleeding	
IV. Laceration	Parenchymal disruption involving 25–50% of hepatic lobe	864.04
V. Laceration	Parenchymal disruption of more than 50% of hepatic lobe	864.14
V. Laceration vascular	Juxtahepatic venous injuries: i.e., retrohepatic vena cava/major hepatic veins	864.14
VI. Vascular	Hepatic avulsion	864.14

Modified with permission from Moore et al. [34, 35].

Table 1. Liver injury scale

Grade	Injury	ICD
I	Contusion or hematoma of the gallbladder	868.02
	Contusion of the portal triad	
II	Partial gallbladder avulsion from liver bed with intact cystic duct	868.02
	Laceration or perforation of the gallbladder	868.12
III	Complete gallbladder avulsion from liver bed	868.02
	Cystic duct laceration	868.12
IV	Partial or complete right hepatic duct laceration	868.12
	Partial or complete left hepatic duct laceration	
	Partial common hepatic duct laceration (<50%)	
	Partial common bile duct laceration (<50%)	
V	Laceration of common hepatic duct (>50%)	868.12
	Laceration of common bile duct (>50%)	
	Combined right and left hepatic duct injuries	
	Intraduodenal or intrahepatic bile duct injuries	

Modified with permission from Moore et al. [34, 35].

Table 2. Extrahepatic biliary tree injury scale.

5.2. Extrahepatic injuries

Extrahepatic bile duct injuries can affect the biliary bifurcation, the hepatic duct, the cystic duct, or the common hepatic duct as summarized in **Table 2**.

6. Management of patients with intrahepatic bile duct injuries

During DCS or subsequent surgeries, ligation or oversewing of the leaking duct is often the only intervention needed. This is usually a relatively straightforward procedure. For patients who are managed conservatively, the natural history of these injuries is spontaneous resolution with scarring of the liver parenchyma and sealing of the bile duct providing that there is no distal bile duct obstruction [36, 37]. However, in a small percentage of patients, bile duct and hepatic parenchyma injuries can cause hemobilia or formation of bilomas.

6.1. Hemobilia

Hemobilia is extravasation of blood in the biliary tree due to the presence of a communication the presence of a communication between a blood vessel and the bile ducts. The majority of symptomatic hemobilias are caused by arterial bleed while hemobilias from venous injuries are quite rare [38]. The frequency of hemobilia after trauma ranges between 3 and 7% [39] with the majority of patients experiencing clinically insignificant and self-limiting blood loss into the biliary tree and in the upper gastrointestinal tract [39]. In these circumstances, arterial blood seeps into the biliary tree and, due to the fibrinolytic activity of the bile, clots rapidly dissolve and often go unnoticed [39]. In a very small proportion of patients, clots might not dissolve and form biliary plugs that can cause biliary obstruction causing jaundice and colic pain [38, 39]. The majority of symptomatic patients with hemobilia present with melena (90%), abdominal pain (70%), and obstructive jaundice (60%) [40, 41]. In trauma, hemobilia should always be suspected when patients present with upper gastrointestinal bleeding since this condition can occur as a late complication [38]. Diagnosis of hemobilia can be confirmed by arterial phase computerized tomography (CT) or selective hepatic artery arteriography. Selective arteriogram by percutaneous approach has become the leading modality to treat hemobilia with microembolization of the arterial branches communicating with the biliary tree with success rates in 84–95% of patients [38, 42]. In the last decade, diagnosis of hemobilia by upper endoscopy has become less frequent as the majority of patients, particularly those with blunt traumas, undergo CT scans that are very sensitive and specific in identifying evidence of active or recent bleeding into the biliary tree and gallbladder by pooling of contrast in the biliary system and presence of intraluminal clots or biliary dilatation [43, 44].

6.2. Bilomas

The rate of liver-related complications in hemodynamically stable patients with blunt traumas is low (0–7%) [45–49]. On the other hand, liver-related complications in high-grade liver injuries are common (11–13%) [49–51]. Ischemic necrosis of the liver and gallbladder, formation of hepatic abscesses, and bile leaks are the most frequent complications of blunt hepatic traumas [52]. Based on clinical signs and symptoms of liver-related complications such as right upper quadrant pain, jaundice, fever, or melena, the optimal time to repeat imaging studies for patients with high-grade liver injuries is usually within 7–10 days [53]. The presence of bilomas is suggested by the progressive growth of a well-circumscribed, low attenuation intraparenchymal or perihepatic fluid collections on cross-sectional imaging studies [54]. The majority of patients with suspected bilomas are currently treated by the placement of percutaneous drainages under radiological guidance while ERCP with the insertion of biliary stenting is indicated for those patients with expanding or persistent bilomas that failed resolution after external drainage [53, 55].

7. Extrahepatic bile duct trauma

7.1. Gallbladder injuries

The gallbladder is relatively protected from blunt traumas due to its anatomic position within the liver parenchyma and behind the ribcage. Similarly, isolated injuries to the gallbladder are uncommon, and mortality is related to other injuries [31, 56, 57]. One of the predisposing factors for both blunt and penetrating trauma to the gallbladder is intraluminal distension. This occurs when secretin and gastrin are released, often after consumption of alcoholic beverages, causing an increasing production of bile and the tone of the sphincter of Oddi. The result is a distended gallbladder and an increased pressure in the biliary tree. When the gallbladder is distended, it becomes less protected by the ribcage and by the liver, and it is more at risk of perforating injuries or blunt forces compressing the gallbladder or decelerations responsible for avulsions.

Traditionally, cholecystectomy has been the recommended treatment for gallbladder injuries with significant contusion or tissue injury [58, 59]. In the past, cholecystorrhaphy was regarded as a risk factor for stone formation and subsequent cholecystitis [60, 61]. However, there is little evidence to support these recommendations, and recently, simple suture repair has been considered acceptable for some patients with minor injuries.

The role of cholecystostomy tubes is very limited and should be avoided due to the increased risk of developing biliary fistulas. However, the placement of a cholecystostomy tube can be useful in the unstable, critically injured patient and might provide access to the biliary tract where there is an associated intrahepatic or distal common bile duct injury [57].

7.2. Common and hepatic duct injuries

The biliary tree is relatively fixed proximally and distally and it does appear that disruption is more prone to occur either at the hilum of the liver or at the junction with the pancreas [21, 61]. When the lesion involves at least 50% of the main bile duct circumference, the majority can be treated by choledochorrhaphy and insertion of a Kehr tube through a different orifice where the biliary duct tissue is healthy. This is a rapid and efficacious technique for trauma

http://dx.doi.org/10.5772/64535

patients who, typically, do not present with dilatation of the bile duct that could facilitate other form of repair. Other techniques using patches to close the defect have been used with variable outcomes. When there is a complete transaction of the bile duct, hepaticojejunostomy is the approach of choice if the patient is hemodynamically stable and there is no frank intra-abdominal contamination. For a selected group of patients who are hemodynamically stable and with scant symptoms, endoscopic sphincterotomy and insertion of biliary prosthesis can be used in addition to percutaneous drainage of concomitant bilomas. The morbidity associated with main bile duct lesions affects approximately 10% of patients who might develop biliary fistulas, hemobilia, bilomas, intrahepatic abscesses, stenosis, and ascending cholangitis. For the majority of patients who die, often the cause of death is unrelated to complications caused by their biliary lesions.

8. Endoscopic management of bile duct injuries

ERCP has become a very attractive diagnostic and treatment modality for patients with extrahepatic biliary trauma. During the ERCP, patients undergo sphincterotomy of the papilla of Vater and cannulation of the common bile duct with placement of a biliary stent to reduce the pressure gradient between the bile duct and the duodenum by eliminating the physiologic role of the sphincter of Oddi. In this way, bile drains preferentially Bile drains preferentially into the duodenum, allowing the disrupted duct to heal spontaneously. The timing of ERCP has been open to debate with some authors suggesting that this should be done as soon as the bile leak is diagnosed. This, however, does not take into consideration the natural history of a bile leak that usually heals, irrespective of the mechanism, provided there is adequate drainage.

9. Natural history of bile duct injuries

Regardless of the type of injury, the natural history of traumas to the biliary tree is spontaneous closure within 3 weeks if the biliary drainage is maintained. Conservative management of bile leaks is safe provided that the patients are adequately drained and remain afebrile.

10. Management of posttraumatic bile duct strictures

Posttraumatic biliary strictures are most likely caused by inflammation and scarring of the involved bile ducts. Traumas induce inflammation that eventually leads to fibrosis and occlusion of the lumen of the involved bile ducts. In addition, the formation of intramural hematomas or direct damage to the arterial supply of the bile duct results in ischemic fibrosis and stricture of the biliary tree. There are very few reports of the incidence and management of posttraumatic bile duct strictures. Previous studies have reported that traumatic bile duct strictures could be managed with percutaneous drainage and/or endoscopic stenting. However, there are no reports on the optimal time for surgical intervention for the repair of late biliary stricture after trauma. Treatment of the bile duct injuries depends on the position and the type of lesions. For an incomplete transection of the common hepatic duct or common bile duct, simple repair over a T-tube or stent is quite appropriate. However, a complete transection where the blood supply of the biliary tract has been disrupted an end-to-end anastomosis should not be performed [62]. In 20 collected cases of traumatic complete transection of the biliary tract repaired by end-to-end anastomosis, the stricture rate requiring reoperation was 55% [61].

11. Conclusions

Noniatrogenic trauma to the extrahepatic biliary tract is uncommon. A high index of suspicion is required for early diagnosis. Most gallbladder injuries are managed by cholecystectomy, with cholecystorrhaphy being reserved only for minor isolated lacerations. Common bile duct injuries are managed by simple repair or biliary-enteric anastomosis depending on whether there is a tangential perforation or a complete transection. Minor bile duct injuries, if symptomatic, can be managed by endoscopic techniques or by interventional radiology modalities. Optimally, these injuries should be managed in specialized hepatobiliary surgery units [57].

Author details

Michele Molinari

Address all correspondence to: michele.molinari@nshealth.ca

1 Dalhousie University, Halifax, Nova Scotia, Canada

2 Department of Surgery Hepatobiliary and Pancreatic Surgery and Transplantation, Dalhousie University, Halifax, Nova Scotia, Canada

References

[1] Rodriguez-Montes JA, Rojo E, Martin LG. Complications following repair of extrahepatic bile duct injuries after blunt abdominal trauma. World J Surg 2001;25:1313–1316.

[2] Stankiewicz R, Najnigier B, Krawczyk M. Is the age of patients with iatrogenic bile duct injuries increasing? Pol Przegl Chir 2015;87:129–133.

[3] Gluszek S, Kot M, Balchanowski N, et al. Iatrogenic bile duct injuries – clinical problems. Pol Przegl Chir 2014;86:17–25.

[4] Addeo P, Saouli AC, Ellero B, et al. Liver transplantation for iatrogenic bile duct injuries sustained during cholecystectomy. Hepatol Int 2013;7:910–915.

[5] Thompson CM, Saad NE, Quazi RR, Darcy MD, Picus DD, Menias CO. Management of iatrogenic bile duct injuries: role of the interventional radiologist. Radiographics 2013;33:117–134.

[6] Jablonska B, Olakowski M, Lampe P, Gorka Z, Buldak L. Quality-of-life assessment in the treatment of iatrogenic bile duct injuries: hepaticojejunostomy versus end-to-end biliary reconstructions. ANZ J Surg 2012;82:923–927.

[7] Dageforde LA, Landman MP, Feurer ID, Poulose B, Pinson CW, Moore DE. A cost-effectiveness analysis of early vs late reconstruction of iatrogenic bile duct injuries. J Am Coll Surg 2012;214:919–927.

[8] Ulitsky A, Werlin S, Dua KS. Role of ERCP in the management of non-iatrogenic traumatic bile duct injuries in the pediatric population. Gastrointest Endosc 2011;73:823–827.

[9] Nuzzo G, Giuliante F, Ardito F, Vellone M, Giovannini I. Re: how to avoid unnecessary laparotomies in iatrogenic bile duct injuries? Am J Surg 2012;203:411.

[10] Jablonska B, Lampe P. Iatrogenic bile duct injuries: etiology, diagnosis and management. World J Gastroenterol 2009;15:4097–4104.

[11] Gronroos JM. How to avoid unnecessary laparotomies in iatrogenic bile duct injuries? Am J Surg 2009;197:133–134.

[12] Parks RW, Spencer EF, McIlrath EM, Johnston GW. A review of the management of iatrogenic bile duct injuries. Ir J Med Sci 1994;163:571–575.

[13] Mishra PK, Saluja SS, Nag HH, Goel N, Jain A, Kujur D. Isolated extrahepatic bile duct injury after blunt trauma abdomen. Am Surg 2012;78:1014–1016.

[14] Balzarotti R, Cimbanassi S, Chiara O, Zabbialini G, Smadja C. Isolated extrahepatic bile duct rupture: a rare consequence of blunt abdominal trauma. Case report and review of the literature. World J Emerg Surg 2012;7:16.

[15] Mirza B, Ijaz L, Iqbal S, Sheikh A. Partial avulsion of common bile duct and duodenal perforation in a blunt abdominal trauma. APSP J Case Rep 2010;1:19.

[16] Agaoglu N. Transection of the common bile duct with partial avulsion of the gallbladder due to blunt trauma. Acta Chir Belg 2009;109:623–625.

[17] Miyayama S, Matsui O, Taki K, et al. Bile duct disruption after blunt hepatic trauma: treatment with percutaneous repair. J Trauma 2006;60:640–643.

[18] Ramia JM, Gutierrez G, Garrote D, Mansilla A, Villar J, Ferron JA. Isolated extrahepatic bile duct rupture in blunt abdominal trauma. Am J Emerg Med 2005;23:231–232.

[19] He Z, Ma K, Sun W, Zhou Y, Gu H. Bile duct injury following blunt abdominal trauma. Chin J Traumatol 2000;3:57–59.

[20] Sofianos C, Naidu M. Complete transection of the common bile duct following blunt abdominal trauma. A case report. S Afr J Surg 1994;32:44–45.

[21] Carmichael DH. Avulsion of the common bile duct by blunt trauma. South Med J 1980;73:166–168.

[22] Ahmed S. Bile duct injuries from non-penetrating abdominal trauma in childhood. Aust N Z J Surg 1976;46:209–212.

[23] Plewes B, McKee JA. Rupture of the common bile duct by blunt trauma. Can Med Assoc J 1968;98:170–171.

[24] Schaer SM, Dziob JM, Brown RK. Bile duct rupture from external blunt trauma. Am J Surg 1955;89:745–747.

[25] van der Wilden GM, Velmahos GC, Emhoff T, et al. Successful nonoperative management of the most severe blunt liver injuries: a multicenter study of the research consortium of new England centers for trauma. Arch Surg 2012;147:423–428.

[26] Navsaria PH, Nicol AJ, Krige JE, Edu S. Selective nonoperative management of liver gunshot injuries. Ann Surg 2009;249:653–656.

[27] Caruso DM, Battistella FD, Owings JT, Lee SL, Samaco RC. Perihepatic packing of major liver injuries: complications and mortality. Arch Surg 1999;134:958–962; discussion 62–63.

[28] Nicol AJ, Hommes M, Primrose R, Navsaria PH, Krige JE. Packing for control of hemorrhage in major liver trauma. World J Surg 2007;31:569–574.

[29] Hollands MJ, Little JM. Non-operative management of blunt liver injuries. Br J Surg 1991;78:968–972.

[30] Hollands MJ, Little JM. Post-traumatic bile fistulae. J Trauma 1991;31:117–120.

[31] Bade PG, Thomson SR, Hirshberg A, Robbs JV. Surgical options in traumatic injury to the extrahepatic biliary tract. Br J Surg 1989;76:256–258.

[32] Hommes M, Nicol AJ, Navsaria PH, Reinders Folmer E, Edu S, Krige JE. Management of biliary complications in 412 patients with liver injuries. J Trauma Acute Care Surg 2014;77:448–451.

[33] Burmeister S, Krige JE, Bornman PC, Nicol AJ, Navsaria P. Endoscopic treatment of persistent thoracobiliary fistulae after penetrating liver trauma. HPB (Oxford) 2009;11:171–175.

[34] Moore EE, Cogbill TH, Jurkovich GJ, Shackford SR, Malangoni MA, Champion HR. Organ injury scaling: spleen and liver (1994 revision). J Trauma 1995;38:323–324.

[35] Moore EE, Jurkovich GJ, Knudson MM, et al. Organ injury scaling. VI: extrahepatic biliary, esophagus, stomach, vulva, vagina, uterus (nonpregnant), uterus (pregnant), fallopian tube, and ovary. J Trauma 1995;39:1069–1070.

[36] Anand RJ, Ferrada PA, Darwin PE, Bochicchio GV, Scalea TM. Endoscopic retrograde cholangiopancreatography is an effective treatment for bile leak after severe liver trauma. J Trauma 2011;71:480–485.

[37] Lucas CE. Endoscopic retrograde cholangiopancreatography for bile leak after severe liver trauma. J Trauma Acute Care Surg 2012;72:537; author reply – 8.

[38] Srivastava DN, Sharma S, Pal S, et al. Transcatheter arterial embolization in the management of hemobilia. Abdom Imaging 2006;31:439–448.

[39] Sandblom P, Saegesser F, Mirkovitch V. Hepatic hemobilia: hemorrhage from the intrahepatic biliary tract, a review. World J Surg 1984;8:41–50.

[40] Yoon W, Jeong YY, Kim JK, et al. CT in blunt liver trauma. Radiographics 2005;25:87–104.

[41] Bloechle C, Izbicki JR, Rashed MY, et al. Hemobilia: presentation, diagnosis, and management. Am J Gastroenterol 1994;89:1537–1540.

[42] Merrell SW, Schneider PD. Hemobilia--evolution of current diagnosis and treatment. West J Med 1991;155:621–625.

[43] Samuels RS, Shriver M, Patel NH. Hemobilia after a gunshot injury to the liver. AJR Am J Roentgenol 1996;166:1304.

[44] Lutter DR, Berger ML. Diagnosis of nontraumatic hematobilia by computerized tomography of the abdomen. Am J Gastroenterol 1988;83:329–330.

[45] Meredith JW, Young JS, Bowling J, Roboussin D. Nonoperative management of blunt hepatic trauma: the exception or the rule? J Trauma 1994;36:529–534; discussion 34–35.

[46] Patton JH, Jr., Croce MA, Fabian TC. Blunt hepatic trauma: trends in nonoperative management. J Tenn Med Assoc 1995;88:101–102.

[47] Velmahos GC, Toutouzas K, Radin R, et al. High success with nonoperative management of blunt hepatic trauma: the liver is a sturdy organ. Arch Surg 2003;138:475–480; discussion 80–81.

[48] Pachter HL, Knudson MM, Esrig B, et al. Status of nonoperative management of blunt hepatic injuries in 1995: a multicenter experience with 404 patients. J Trauma 1996;40:31–38.

[49] Malhotra AK, Fabian TC, Croce MA, et al. Blunt hepatic injury: a paradigm shift from operative to nonoperative management in the 1990s. Ann Surg 2000;231:804–813.

[50] Pachter HL, Feliciano DV. Complex hepatic injuries. Surg Clin North Am 1996;76:763–782.

[51] Kozar RA, Moore FA, Cothren CC, et al. Risk factors for hepatic morbidity following nonoperative management: multicenter study. Arch Surg 2006;141:451–458; discussion 8–9.

[52] Mohr AM, Lavery RF, Barone A, et al. Angiographic embolization for liver injuries: low mortality, high morbidity. J Trauma 2003;55:1077–1081; discussion 81–82.

[53] Bala M, Gazalla SA, Faroja M, et al. Complications of high grade liver injuries: management and outcomewith focus on bile leaks. Scand J Trauma Resusc Emerg Med 2012;20:20.

[54] De Backer A, Fierens H, De Schepper A, Pelckmans P, Jorens PG, Vaneerdeweg W. Diagnosis and nonsurgical management of bile leak complicated by biloma after blunt liver injury: report of two cases. Eur Radiol 1998;8:1619–1622.

[55] Marks JM, Ponsky JL, Shillingstad RB, Singh J. Biliary stenting is more effective than sphincterotomy in the resolution of biliary leaks. Surg Endosc 1998;12:327–330.

[56] Hirshberg A, Thomson SR, Bade PG, Huizinga WK. Pitfalls in the management of penetrating chest trauma. Am J Surg 1989;157:372–375; discussion 6.

[57] Hills MW, Richardson AJ, Tait N, Deane SA, Little JM. Non-iatrogenic trauma to the extrahepatic biliary tract. Aust N Z J Surg 1993;63:190–194.

[58] Posner MC, Moore EE. Extrahepatic biliary tract injury: operative management plan. J Trauma 1985;25:833–837.

[59] Kitahama A, Elliott LF, Overby JL, Webb WR. The extrahepatic biliary tract injury: perspective in diagnosis and treatment. Ann Surg 1982;196:536–540.

[60] Feliciano DV, Bitondo CG, Burch JM, Mattox KL, Beall AC, Jr., Jordan GL, Jr. Management of traumatic injuries to the extrahepatic biliary ducts. Am J Surg 1985;150:705–709.

[61] Ivatury RR, Rohman M, Nallathambi M, Rao PM, Gunduz Y, Stahl WM. The morbidity of injuries of the extra-hepatic biliary system. J Trauma 1985;25:967–973.

[62] Northover JM, Terblanche J. A new look at the arterial supply of the bile duct in man and its surgical implications. Br J Surg 1979;66:379–384.

Chapter 9

Liver Trauma

Marco Massani, Luca Bonariol, Bruno Pauletti,
Cesare Ruffolo, Roberta Bonariol,
Ezio Caratozzolo and Nicolo' Bassi

Additional information is available at the end of the chapter

http://dx.doi.org/10.5772/64543

Abstract

Objective: The aim of this section is to assess the evolution in the management of liver injuries during the last two decades.

Methods: The authors reviewed the English literature, reporting the wider experiences, and on the basis of the personal experience, they suggest an up to date treatment.

Results: Mortality due to hepatic injury has decreased over the past century from nearly 70% at the beginning of last century to the current level of 6–7%. This could be partially attributed to the improvement of operative techniques, to a lower surgical trend, to the application of damage control laparotomy in very complex liver trauma, and particularly to the diffusion of hepatic angiographic embolization. Scientific evidence has shown that more than 67% of laparotomies performed for blunt liver trauma are not therapeutic and in about 86% of all post-traumatic hepatic lesions the hemorrhage stopped spontaneously at the time of the laparotomy. On the other hand, blunt hepatic trauma can be conservatively treated in 70–90% of hemodynamic stable patients, in the absence of other associated lesions/peritoneal signs or in the case of limited need for transfusions. Thus far, the main decision criteria for a surgical rather than a conservative approach to the management of liver trauma have been the hemodynamic stability and not the American Association for the Surgery of Trauma-Organ Injury Scale (AAST-OIS) grading of the lesion.

Conclusions: Restricting the indications for a conservative treatment of liver traumas solely to the relief of hemodynamic stability seems nowadays to be unreasonable. Criteria for a conservative treatment are as follows: hemodynamic stability, limited need of blood transfusions, and non-associated visceral lesions on CT scan. In the presence of these conditions non-operative approach can be undertaken, and the cornerstone of this treatment is transarterial angiographic embolization.

Keywords: Liver trauma, embolization, laparotomy, interventional radiology, associated lesions

1. Objective

Liver and spleen are the most frequently injured organs in blunt abdominal trauma. Management of hepatic trauma has nowadays radically changed in comparison with the past, when the chance of spontaneous hemostasis of hepatic lacerations was considered an impossible event, and conservative management appeared dangerous. Therefore, surgery was almost ever the best therapeutic option for the patient with liver injury. In the 1980s–1990s, surgical indication for liver trauma was dictated not only by the need to control hemorrhage or control biliary leak, but also to reveal concomitant unknown hollow viscus injuries. At the beginning of twentieth century, most hepatic injuries had fatal outcome, despite the routinely use of liver pedicle clamping introduced by J. Hogarth Pringle in 1908.

2. Methods

The authors reviewed the English literature, reporting the wider experience in the management of liver trauma and considering their personal experience; during 20 years, they analyzed how liver trauma management has changed in the last two decade.

3. Results

Nowadays, mortality for hepatic injury has decreased significantly as reported in the analysis of data collected by the National Trauma Data Bank (NTDB) (under the aegis of the American College of Surgeons Committee on Trauma NTDB (2008)) from nearly 70% at the beginning of last century to 16.7% between 2000 and 2004 [1]. Current series report a mortality rate of 6–7% for liver trauma [2].

Many factors led to decrease mortality rate, including:

- better knowledge of liver physiopathology,
- non-operative management (NOM) (success rate of 80–90%),
- development of high experience centers in hepatobiliary surgery,
- damage control laparotomy (DCL) in complex liver trauma.

Moreover, new CT scan techniques can provide more detailed images of hepatic lesions, exclude hollow viscus injuries and quantify the amount of blood into peritoneal cavity.

http://dx.doi.org/10.5772/64543

These factors have drastically changed the approach to liver trauma, which is no longer an exclusive dominion of the surgeons.

3.1. Classification

Liver injury is often due to a polytrauma; therefore, its management needs a score to state severity of clinical condition: frequently adopted scales are Revised Trauma Score (RTS) and Injury Severity Score (ISS).

Liver	Abbreviated Injury Scale Score (AIS)
Grade I	2
Hematoma: sub capsular, < 10% surface area	2
Laceration : capsular tear, < 1 cm parenchymal depth	
Grade II	2
Hematoma: subcapsular, 10% to 50% surface area, intraparenchymal < 10 cm in diameter	2
Laceration: capsular tear 1 to 3 cm parenchymal depth, < 10 cm in length	
Grade III	3
Hematoma: subcapsular, > 50% surface area, ruptured subcapsular or parenchymal hematoma; intraparenchymal hematoma >10 cm or expanding	3
Laceration: >3 cm parenchymal depth	
Grade IV	4
Laceration: parenchymal disruption involving 25% to 75% hepatic lobe or 1 to 3 Coinaud's segments	
Grade V	5
Laceration: parenchymal disruption involving > 75% of hepatic lobe or > 3 Coinaud's segments within a single lobe	5
Vascular: juxtahepatic venous injuries, ie retrohepatic vena cava/central major hepatic vein	
Grade VI	6
Vascular hepatic avulsion	

Table 1. Liver Injury classification according to American association for the Surgery of Trauma-Organ Injury Scale.

Revised Trauma Score (RTS) is based on three parameters: blood pressure, breathing, and Glasgow Coma Scale (GCS) each of them is quantified with a level score from 0 to 4. A cumulative score <11 is considered as a severe condition [3].

On the contrary, ISS is a more complex scoring system generally closely related to morbidity, mortality, and length of hospital stay. It is based on Abbreviated Injury Scale (AIS) that assigned a six-grade score for each of six body regions. The score ranges between 1 and 25; thus, the trauma is considered mild for score <9, moderate for 10–14, and severe for 15–24 [4].

Both previous reported score systems are useful for evaluating trauma in its complexity but in order to create an injury severity scale for single organs; in 1987, the American Association for the Surgery of Trauma (AAST) assessed the Organ Injury Scale (OIS), which is now the most frequently adopted [5] (**Table 1**). The scale, first proposed by Moore and revised in 1994, includes six grades of severity.

Based on Moore classification, Mirvis scale was designed on CT scan findings (**Table 2**) [6]. OIS-AAST grading system provides a descriptive value of hepatic injury, but its utility in clinical practice is somehow limited, because it does not correlate with specific treatment of the hepatic trauma.

Recently, the National Trauma Data Bank (NTDB) [2] under the aegis of the American College for Surgeons Committee on Trauma tried to give a clinical value to the AAST-OIS scale.

The NTDB V. 5.0 included 1,130,093 patients from 405 centers in USA between 2000 and 2004 with liver, kidney, and spleen trauma, isolated or associated with other lesions. Data analysis showed that mortality rate increased as well as grade of lesions: for patients with liver trauma, grade 1–2 associated with other lesions was reported a mortality of 12.7%, 15% for grade 3, 27.9% for grade 4, 64.8 % for grade 5, and 94.9% for grade 6.

Overall mortality was 16.7%, and 80–90% of patients with hepatic and kidney trauma had undergone NOM. Nevertheless, operative rate increased as well as grading from 29.2 to 37.2%.

Grade	
1	Capsular avulsion, superficial laceration (s) <1cm deep, subcapsular hematoma <1 cm maximal thickness, periportal blood tracking only
2	Lacerations (s) 1–3 cm deep, central/subcapsular hematoma (s) 1–3 cm in diameter
3	Lacerations (s) > 3 cm deep, , central/subcapsular hematoma (s) >3 cm in diameter
4	Massive central/subcapsular hematoma (s) >10 cm in diameter, lobar tissue destruction (maceration) or devascularization
5	Bilobar tissue destruction (maceration) or devascularization

Table 2. Mirvis classification of liver trauma (Mirvis).

3.2. Non-operative Management (NOM)

Since 1990, management of liver trauma has become more and more conservative, particularly due to studies on pediatric population. Karp et al. reported 17 pediatric cases with blunt hepatic trauma successfully managed without surgical intervention. Moreover, he described four stages of damaged liver healing: (1) blood reabsorbtion within the first 2 weeks, (2) coalescence of the laceration, (3) size reduction, and (4) restitutio ad integrum in a period of 3–4 months [7]. Furthermore, reviewing CT scans, he revealed that 20–67% of laparotomies for trauma were not therapeutic and in 50–85% of hepatic lacerations, bleeding has already stopped at the moment of surgical exploration [8].

Results from pediatric experience gained considerable popularity also in adult trauma management, and around 1995–1996 first reports about NOM appeared in literature, even if they concern small series and not uniform population. However, success rate of conservative treatment has been reported between 17 and 60%.

In a prospective study by Malhotra et al., a population of 661 patients with blunt trauma was compared to other two patient cohorts of previous years (1985–1990 and 1993–1994); starting from this analysis, a new "paradigm shift" of liver trauma management in non-operative approach was provided [9]. Success rate of conservative management was 92.5%, associated with a low rate of intra-abdominal infections, low need of blood transfusions, and shorter hospital stay. Failure of NOM was due to hepatic-related causes in only 48% of cases.

The early studies about NOM were performed on patients with low grade lesions (I-II AAST-OIS) and reported a success rate of conservative management around 70–90% [10]. More recent experience showed good results also in stable patients with grade 4–5 liver injuries.

A recent analysis of NTDB V. 5.0 (between 2000 and 2004) [2] that tried to validate the AAST-OIS, showed that only 14% of patients with liver trauma needs surgical operation, and in case of isolated hepatic trauma, success rate of NOM was, respectively, 91.5% for grade 1–2 lesions, 79% for grade 3, 72.8% for grade 4, and 62.6% for grade 5.

The same results were described by Hurtuk et al. [11], reporting a success rate of 76.6, 69.3, and 62.3%, respectively, for grades 3, 4, and 5 lesions, and by Polanco et al. [12] in recent review of 3627 patients with blunt liver trauma and AAST-OIS score ≥4, reporting a success rate of NOM >90%.

On the contrary, Kozar et al. [13] reported a success rate of 40% in grade 4 injuries and only 4% in grade 5.

Finally, in multicentre retrospective study including 393 patients with blunt liver trauma AAST-OIS grade 4–5, the authors confirmed good results with NOM even in complex liver injuries. Two-thirds of patients underwent conservative treatment with a success rate of 91.3% [14].

Therefore, the lesson from these studies is that NOM is considered advisable even for severe hepatic injuries, assuming that hemodynamic stability is verified (**Figures 1** and **2**).

It should be noted that even if the shift towards non-operative management drastically improved survival of patients with hepatic trauma, its high success rate does not release surgeon from close supervision, especially in patients with complex liver injuries. Richardson [1] reported that mortality for liver trauma decreased from 19 to 9% in a 25 years lapse and liver directly related death from 12 to 5% not only for the introduction of non-operative management of grade 4–5 liver trauma, but also due to improvement in surgical techniques and use of damage control laparotomy.

The most important selection criteria for a conservative approach to patients with hepatic trauma are in summary:

- hemodynamic stability (blood pressure ≥90 mm Hg and good response after fluid resuscitation),
- limited need of blood transfusions (≤4 UI/24 h),
- non-associated visceral lesions on CT scan.

In the presence of these conditions non-operative approach can be undertaken, and the cornerstone of this treatment is transarterial angiographic embolization.

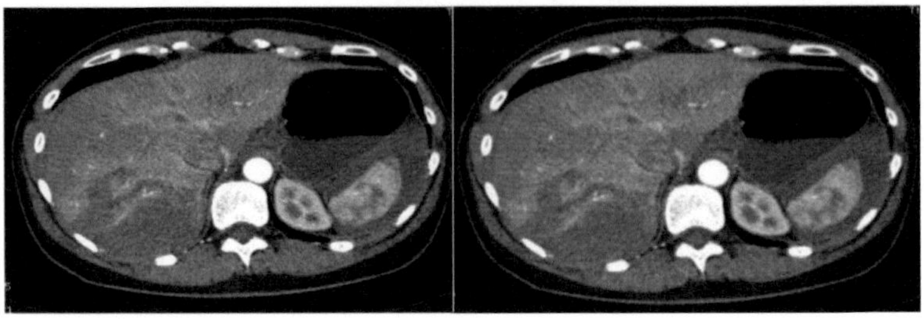

Figure 1. Female, 49 years old, cyclist hit by a truck. She was hemodynamically stable, blood pressure 110/80 mmHg, RTS 12, hemoglobin 12 gr/dl, GCS 15. CT scan of abdomen and chest was performed at admission with evidence of pneumothorax and multiple lacerations in the right lobe of the liver, Mirvis scale grade 3–4, with hemoperitoneum, but not vascular blush. She was not transfused and conservatively treated. Discharged after 15 days in good health.

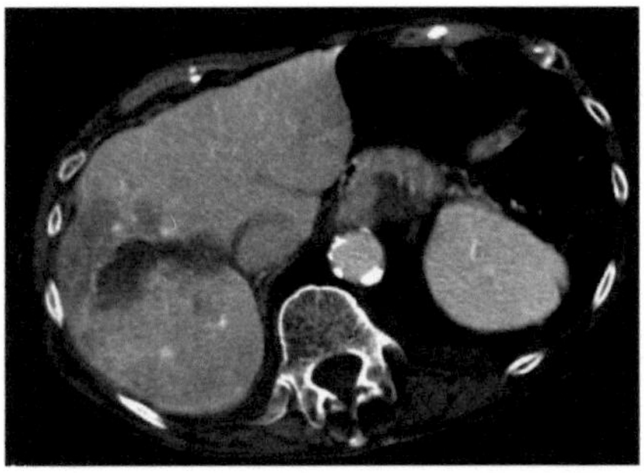

Figure 2. Female, 91 years old, with chest trauma following accidentally fall in her house. Ct scan showed deep laceration in the central part of the liver, Mirvis scale grade 3. The patient was conservatively treated with success and discharged after 13 days.

3.2.1. Transarterial angiographic embolization (TAE)

The introduction in clinical practice of angiographic embolization, based on CT scan finding of contrast blush, is the factor that most contributed to improvement in survival.

Arterial hemorrhage differs from venous bleeding because it cannot be stopped by simple manual compression or by packing. Thus, use of angiographic embolization has increased both in NOM and after damage control laparotomy.

http://dx.doi.org/10.5772/64543

A recent review of our experience concerning the treatment of grade 3–4 hepatic trauma revealed that since 2005, thanks to the introduction of a new, high quality multislice CT scanner and to greater improvement in angiographic embolization expertise, the success rate of NOM has significantly increased compared to the past, with lower conversion to laparotomy (6% vs 62%) and operative rate (52% vs 22%) [15].

Fang et al. [16] divided the CT finding of contrast blush into three groups:

- free extravasation into peritoneal cavity;
- intraparenchymal bleeding with concomitant hemoperitoneum;
- intraparenchymal contrast blush without hemoperitoneum.

Intraperitoneal contrast extravasation, in presence of hemodynamic stability, is considered a strong indication for early angiographic embolization, and it is, however, an independent predictive factor for the need of operative treatment.

It is quite controversial whether to perform angiographic embolization in hemodynamically stable patients presenting intraparenchymal blush rather than submit them to close observation, performing angiographic embolization only in cases of remarkable signs of bleeding.

Moreover, contrast blush detected at CT scan is not always confirmed by subsequent angiography. This is another interesting aspect because it is still debated whether to continue with embolization anyway, taking the risk of hepatic ischemia, rather than stop the procedure and start a close monitoring as soon as the first signs of hemorrhage appear. A recent study by Alarhayem et al. [17] reported 68 patients with Ct scan evidence of contrast blush; 22 (33%) of them had no sign of contrast pooling at subsequent angiography and therefore did not undergo embolization. The re-bleeding rate in this group was 32%, significantly higher than what observed in embolized patients. According to the authors, patients should undergo angioembolization procedures when clear CT scan signs of contrast blush are visible.

The same results were reported by Hagiwara et al. [18] comparing CT scan to angiography in detecting contrast extravasation.

The Eastern Association for the Surgery of trauma guidelines assign a level 2 recommendation for angioembolization in hemodynamically stable patients with contrast blush evidence on abdominal CT scan [19] (**Figures 3** and **4a–c**).

A challenging issue proposed by some authors is the use of angioembolization in high-grade hepatic injury found radiologic, despite the finding of contrast blush.

Poletti et al. [20] compared CT scan to angiography in 72 patients with blunt hepatic trauma. The author took into consideration hepatic injury, with or without major veins involvement (the first group had a bleeding risk 3.5 times higher). According to the authors' experience, angiography should routinely be performed in all patients with grade 4 liver trauma when hepatic major veins are involved.

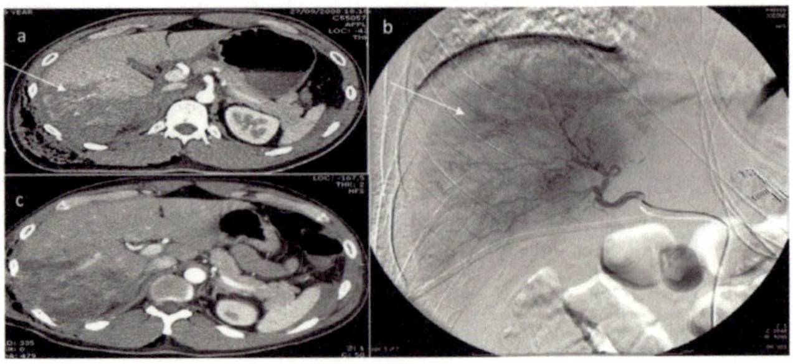

Figure 3. Male, 29 years old, admtted in emergency department for abdominal and chest trauma following fall with paragliding. GCS 15, RTS 12, hemodynamically stable. (a) Ct scan showed deep lacerations in the right liver, large hemoperitoneum and extraparenchymal vascular blush. (b) The patient underwent angiography with evidence of blush in the lateral segments of the liver and selective embolization was performed with gelfoam. (c) CT scan at 48 h. The hospital stay was uneventful and the patient was not trasfused.

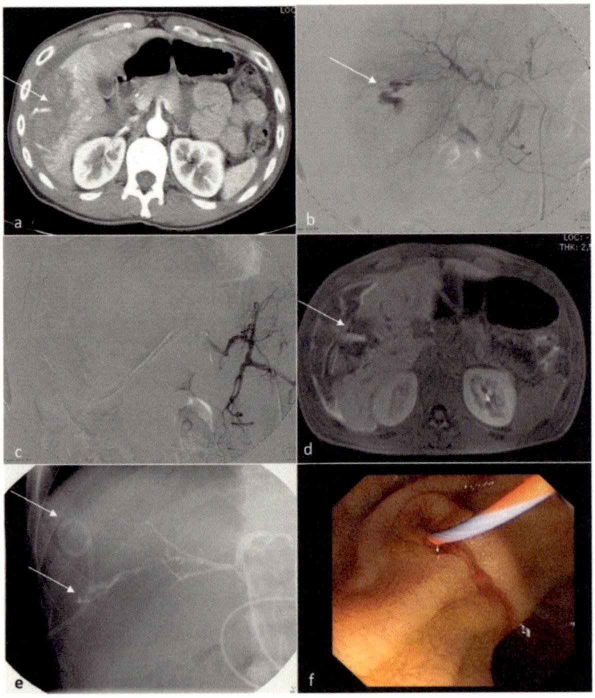

Figure 4. Carpenter, 35 years old hit by a piece of wood in his abdomen. At admission CT scan (a) revealed large hemo peritoneum due to deep lacerations in 5-6 segments of the liver with vascular blush. He underwent angiography (b) that confirmed the blush originating from branch of the right hepatic artery for the fifth segment. The patient was embolized with gelfoam in the distal part of the right hepatic artery and metal coils. No evidence of blush at the end of the procedure (c). In the followings days the patients remained always stable, but he developed jaundice. An MRI (d) was performed that showed deep no bleeding laceration in the lateral segments of the liver, large perihepatic biliary collection with biliary fistula due to traumatic disruption of the dilated biliary ducts inside the laceration (e). The fluid collection was drained by percutaneously insertion of pig-tail (e), and the biliary fistula healed after ERCP and stent insertion (f).

Carrillo [21] reported a 83% efficacy rate in arterial hemorrhage control in liver trauma, whereas Sirivrikoz [22] demonstrated that angiographic embolization is an independent survival factor (AOR 0.48, 95% CI; 36–63, $p < 0.01$) in a series of 6042 patients with isolated grade 4-5 hepatic trauma (years 2002–2011, NTDB. multivariate analysis). In another multi-center study [14], TAE was administered to the two-thirds of patients with grade 4–5 hepatic trauma, with a 91.3% success rate; a quarter of them had undergone angioembolization.

Angioembolization efficacy in hepatic trauma has so far widely been confirmed. Nevertheless, this procedure is not free from life-threatening complications. Hepatic necrosis, gallbladder ischemia, biliary fistulas, and hepatic abscess have been well described in the literature, with a morbidity rate that varies from 29 to 80% [23]. In 2003, Mohr et al. [24] reported a considerably high incidence of complications in patients with hepatic trauma treated by embolization, with a gallbladder infarction rate of 15%.

Letoublon et al. described a 70% morbidity rate in 23 patients treated with TAE [25]. According to the author, however, complications are not exclusively caused by the procedure itself, but also a consequence of complexity of liver trauma.

Dabbs [26] reported a post-TAE hepatic necrosis rate of 42%. TAE morbidity rate is variable and complications are more often caused by the severity of liver trauma than by the procedure itself, which should definitely be performed in selected patients in order to avoid specific hepatic complications.

From 1993 to 2015, 222 patients with hepatic trauma were referred to our Institution; 43% of them have been submitted to NOM. In our experience, we noticed that after 2005, with the introduction of a new, high-quality multislice CT scan and the improvement in angiographic arterial embolization procedures, 70% of patients with grade ≥3 AAST-OIS hepatic trauma underwent NOM with a success rate of 91%. Seventeen (26%) hemodynamically stable patients underwent TAE for contrast extravasation revealed at CT scan. Three patients with severe hepatic trauma underwent TAE even in the absence of bleeding at CT scan, but confirmed at angiographic images. One patient underwent embolization after damage control laparotomy. Two patients were submitted to laparotomy for gallbladder infarction and coleperitoneum. Efficacy, morbidity and mortality rate of TAE were 100, 53 and 18%, respectively. Just in one case, a complication (gallbladder infarction) was directly caused by the procedure.

3.2.2. Prognostic factors

The success of conservative management in blunt liver trauma is related to the ability to predict the need for surgical intervention before deterioration of patients' clinical conditions. Conservative approach may sometimes lead to late hemodynamic instability and the need of an emergent laparotomy, with increased surgical risks; In fact, operations performed in critical conditions when patient's parameters have worsened is certainly more challenging.

Some reports provide that negative prognostic factors at admission are blood pressure <110 mmHg and base deficit of 4 [26, 27]. Almost 25% of patients with liver trauma conservatively treated, need a surgical intervention for complications or NOM failure and in the 3.1–6.7% of cases there is the possibility to ignore concomitant hollow viscus injuries [28]. Furthermore, failure of NOM is associated with increased mortality, particularly in high-grade trauma [12]. This implies that a critical approach and intensive surveillance for patients with hepatic lesions grade ≥3–4 conservatively treated is mandatory, especially if hypotensive at admission and with high ISS.

According to Malhotra et al. [9], bad hemodynamic parameters at admission, high ISS, large hemoperitoneum, and vascular blush on CT scan represent risk factors for NOM failure, even if none of them have a predictive value in statistical terms.

Polanco et al. [12] reported others risk factors as age (OR 1.02), male gender (OR 1.73), high ISS (OR 1.02), low GCS, and low blood pressure at admission (OR 2.07).

A recent systematic review of the literature considered eight prospective studies including 410 patients. Failure of NOM was observed in 9.5% of cases, mortality rate was 4%, and 26 prognostic factors were identified, even if only six of them had a statistical relevance: blood pressure, fluid resuscitation, blood transfusion, the presence of peritoneal signs, ISS and intra-abdominal-associated lesions. Grading of hepatic trauma was not considered a risk factor for NOM failure [29].

In the absence of specific criteria to certainly predict which patients with blunt hepatic trauma would develop hemodynamic instability or complications after NOM, Fang et al. [30] identified some CT scan findings that can predict thc need of surgical operation:

- intraperitoneal contrast blush, hemoperitoneum involving six abdominal compartments,
- hepatic trauma involving more than two segments,
- high-grade Mirvis scale,
- porta hepatis involvement, hepatic lacerations depth >6 cm.

Among them, only intraperitoneal contrast blush, and hemoperitoneum involving six abdominal compartments result predictive factors at multivariate analysis.

3.2.3. NOM failure and complications

Approximately 25–27% of hepatic trauma conservatively treated needs a surgical intervention for complication or late hemorrhage [31]. Therefore, non-operative management of hepatic trauma should be considered not only in terms of mortality but also in terms of morbidity: Overall morbidity is about 0–7% but can be higher than 14% in high-grade lesions. Kozar et al. [32] analyzed 699 patients with blunt liver trauma grade 3–5. About 65% of them was conservatively treated, and they reported an overall morbidity of 14%. Complications including bleeding, bile leaks, infections, and abdominal compartment syndrome (ACS) were reported in 5% of grade 3 lesions, 22% of grade 4, and 52% of grade 5. ACS and bleeding were the most common complications during the first days, while after the third day, patients presented biliary and infectious complications more frequently. At multivariate analysis, grading, and transfusion number within 24 h were predictive factors for complications occurrence.

Management of complication after NOM, recognized on CT scan, should be multimodal, especially in case of biliary accidents as biloma, biliary fistula, and biliary peritonitis. Such kind of problems occur in 3% of cases, particularly in grade 4 lesions, and represent one-third of liver-related complications (**Figure 4d–e**) [27].

Small bilomas usually undergo radiologic observation, and in case of increasing in size, a percutaneous drainage placed under ultrasonography control may be required (**Figure 4e**). ERCP and stenting are the most common techniques in case of major biliary fistula (**Figure 4f**). In case of biliary peritonitis with systemic signs of inflammatory reaction, a laparotomy or laparoscopy with multiple drainages placement and hepatic resectional debridement may be necessary. Bleeding complications usually occur within 72 h after trauma and can be successfully controlled with angiographic embolization in most of cases, even in sometimes a surgical intervention is mandatory.

3.2.4. Follow-up in NOM

It is by now well demonstrated that patients with complex liver trauma must be carefully monitored in Intensive Care Unit (ICU).

On the contrary, the indication to radiologic follow-up during hospital stay and after discharge is still controversial. In a multicentre study, Patcher et al. [33] assert that there is no indication for CT scan follow-up for patients with grade 1–3 liver trauma. The same results are reported by Carrillo et al. [34] while they suggest a radiologic observation for patients with severe hepatic trauma (grades 4–5) when precise conditions (hemodynamic abnormalities, abdominal pain, drop of hemoglobin level, and increase of liver function tests) are revealed.

It is well known that healing time of hepatic injuries, as shown by CT scan observation, is 4–12 weeks; therefore, these patients may resume their physical activity after at least 4 weeks in case of grade 1–3 injuries and after 8 weeks for grade 4–5 injuries.

Cox et al. [35] showed that at CT scan control, 86% of patients presents no modification in liver lesions within the first week after trauma. An improvement was seen between 7 and 10 days after injury and an almost complete healing after 3 months.

3.3. Operative treatment

In the era of interventional radiology, non-operative treatment has become the most used approach in liver blunt trauma. Nevertheless, up to 35% of patients with complex hepatic injury (12–15% of all hepatic injuries) still needs surgical treatment [23, 36–38].

Forty years ago, all patients with liver injury underwent surgical exploration, because liver parenchyma was considered unsuitable for spontaneous hemostasis, and mortality rate exceeded 80% [36, 39].

Starting from the second half of the last century, the introduction of NOM and use of arterial embolization and the improvement of surgical strategies and surgeons ability have radically changed prognosis of these patients [40].

Indeed, the main indications for early surgical exploration in blunt abdominal trauma are by now hemodynamic instability with hemoperitoneum and the presence of peritonitis (in most of cases, it concerns grade 4 and 5 lesions). Patient with low blood pressure, not responding to fluid resuscitation should undergo urgent laparotomy [23, 41, 42]. In this context, well known that the choice of the correct strategy is essential to influence the final outcome of the patient. Critical decision-making, profound knowledge of liver anatomy, and surgical expertise in liver surgery are crucial points, and for these reasons, the operation should be managed by a dedicated liver team [36, 37, 41].

A correct approach must be systematic (**Figure 5**) and follows some "gold rules": use simple maneuvers, pack and compress the liver for damage control, stop the operation when patient is stable, and postpone adjunctive procedure to a second look [39, 41, 43]. This is the concept of "damage control surgery," introduced by Stone at al. in 1980s and promulgated by many authors in numerous large group studies [38, 39, 41, 42].

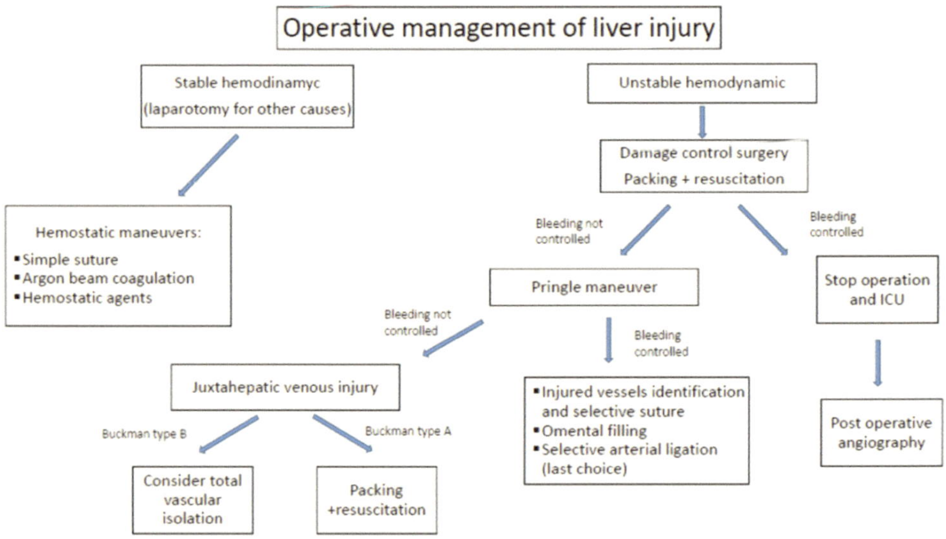

Figure 5. Flowchart for operative management of liver trauma.

Laparotomy should nearly always start with a midline incision with adequate exposure of the upper abdomen. In case of a complex right lobe injury or vena cava lesion, a right extension of the incision may be necessary. Rarely, a sternotomy is needed to control a lesion of the inferior vena cava (IVC) [37, 43].

The initial maneuvers are essential and are directed to control bleeding and allow resuscitation and must be simple and determined [37]. The liver should be manually compressed pushing both the lobe in their natural position and toward the diaphragm. This procedure can stop venous bleeding and allows intra-operative resuscitation. This is a crucial phase, because a delay in control of hemorrhage could lead to the "triad of death": hypothermia, acidosis, and coagulopathy; this is a high-risk condition for patient death. For this reason, it is recommended

http://dx.doi.org/10.5772/64543

to use damage control surgery as a routine procedure and not as the last desperate option when other maneuvers for bleeding control have failed and the situation is deteriorating [37–39, 42].

An early damage control leads to survival of up to 67% of patients, versus only 2% when used as an extreme ratio [36].

Surgical strategy of damage control includes packing technique: Folded laparotomy packs are inserted around the liver, pushing it posteriorly against diaphragmatic surface; some authors suggested to take down the falciform ligament, even if it is a debatable maneuver (**Figure 6**) [23]. Packing must be performed correctly, because a wrong pads positioning could worsen hemorrhage: it is important not to place pads within the liver injury and avoid to pack so tightly that inferior vena cava could be compressed and venous return impaired [23, 36, 37, 43].

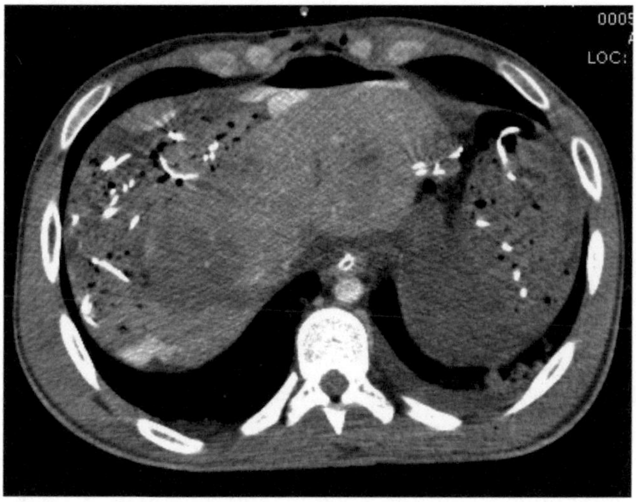

Figure 6. CT scan after damage control surgery.

If these maneuvers prove to be effective, the operation should be stopped and the patient taken to intensive care unit, where a close observation can be performed.

Perihepatic packing can completely control low pressure bleeding, originated from portal and hepatic veins, but it is not resolutive for arterial bleeding. For this reasons, many authors suggest the use of postoperative angiography and eventual selective embolization after damage control surgery because more than 50% of patients demonstrate bleeding at postoperative radiographic control. Even if prospective studies are needed, arterial embolization should be incorporated in the management of bleeding after perihepatic packing [38, 42, 43]. Intra-operative selective ligation of hepatic artery should be avoided for the high risk of parenchymal and gallbladder necrosis and reserved for selective cases of massive uncontrollable bleeding [38, 40, 43].

Once the physiologic status of the patients has been restored, packing removal can be considered. The optimal timing of pads removal is still controversial, but it is evident that if performed before 24 h, risk of re-bleeding is very high. On the other hand, packing removal after 72 h increases risk of sepsis; even if not yet well defined, 48 h seem to be the best time for second look [36, 37, 40].

If bleeding persists after damage control procedures, Pringle maneuver should be applied placing an atraumatic clamp, or preferably a double vessel loop, around the liver pedicle. This can control bleeding from hepatic artery or portal vein; if hemorrhage persists after hilar clamp, a juxtahepatic venous injury should be suspected [37].

Pringle maneuver must be intermittent, clamping the porta hepatis for 10–15 min and taking it off for 5 min, to avoid parenchymal ischemic suffering and postoperative liver failure [43].

Once bleeding is controlled, injured vessels and bile ducts must be identified and sutured. It is suitable to avoid deep rough suture, especially in profound lesions, for the high risk of main vessel ligations, abscess and hematomas/bilomas formations, and late bleeding. It is advisable to identify the injured structures and selectively repair them; to allow this maneuver, it could be necessary to extend the parenchymal lesion using the finger fracture technique or sometimes a stapling device [37, 43].

To control the hemorrhage, Stone and Lamb proposed the insertion of a viable omental pedicle into the parenchymal injury. It seems to have an effective hemostatic effect, filling the "dead space" with vascularized tissue, introducing peritoneal macrophages into a potential area of sepsis, and providing stromal cell-derived factor 1-alpha which may recruits chemokine receptor cells vital for healing [36, 38].

An issue that in the last years raised great discussions is the role of liver resection in the management of hepatic trauma. Advances in operative techniques lead to decrease mortality for liver resection from 80% in 1900 to less than 20% [37, 38]. Moreover, anatomic resection of an injured segment definitively controls bleeding and potential bile leak and removes devitalized tissue; however, its employment is still controversial.

Polanco et al. reported in a great series of liver resection for liver trauma a mortality lower than 9% and morbidity lower than 30% [39, 44].

Some authors assert that the majority of liver resections performed for hepatic trauma can be considered as resectional debridements of destroyed parenchyma rather than formal hepatic resection [39].

Therefore, simple maneuvers with packing and damage control are the treatment of choice, and the recourse to liver resections must be considered when simple methods fail to successfully control parenchymal bleeding and should, however, be performed by expert liver surgeons.

Finally, hepatic resection can be evaluated at re-exploration to remove injured or necrotic parenchyma as definitive treatment [37, 39, 43].

Juxtahepatic venous injury (grade 5 lesions) represents the most challenging and most deadly form of liver trauma, even if it is a rare event. The patients may be stable and, in rare cases, treated non-operatively, but 92% of them needs urgent operation. The mortality rate described is between 33 and 81%, mainly due to the surgical inaccessible location of the retrohepatic vena cava or hepatic veins [37, 45].

Buckman et al. [46] described two types of iuxtahepatic lesions: Type A includes lesions of the intraparenchymal tract of hepatic veins, usually associated with tissue disruption, most often involving the central posterior portion of the liver. This is the most common lesion and hemorrhage is well controlled in most of cases with perihepatic packing or simple suturing. It is not advisable to mobilize the liver and expose hepatic veins to perform a direct repair of the vessels, for the high risk of bleeding worsening [36, 38, 43, 46].

The second pattern, type B, is represented by extra-parenchymal venous lesion, and it is frequently associated to disruption of suspensory ligaments of the liver or diaphragm. It often leads to an uncontained hemorrhage and may require total vascular isolation by clamping inferior vena cava above and under the liver. In this case, mobilization of the liver is mandatory, and it may be necessary to extend incisions cutting the diaphragm to achieve a correct exposure of the injured vessel. Venovenous bypass or atriocava shunt are not advisable in the management of these injuries [36–38, 46].

Liver transplantation may be an option in rare cases when there is a lesion of the main portal triad structure that cannot be repaired (grade 6 lesion), or in the presence of an uncontrollable bleeding despite the use of all the procedures described above. A further indication can be postoperative liver acute failure [36, 41, 43].

3.4. Operative treatment complications

Complications of surgical treatment of liver trauma include parenchymal necrosis with hepatic abscess, sepsis, re-bleeding, and bile leakage [41, 47].

Re-starting of hemorrhage should possibly be treated with angiography and arterial embolization, rather than ad adjunctive surgical intervention.

If bile leakage and biloma are present, less invasive procedure as ERCP or radiologic drainage is the first choice, unless it may occur a peritonitis for choleperitoneum that requires re-laparotomy [41].

Parenchymal necrosis is a less frequent complication and occurs when a destroyed parenchyma is left in situ after damage control, but can be related to a deep suture closing important vessels, or to hepatic artery ligation/embolization. It can be treated non-operatively, but sometimes, an abscess can develop, and a percutaneous or surgical drainage is necessary [41, 47].

4. Conclusions

Scientific evidence has shown that more than 67% of laparotomies performed for blunt liver trauma are not therapeutic and in about 86% of all post-traumatic hepatic lesions the hemorrhage stopped spontaneously at the time of the laparotomy itself. By contrast, blunt hepatic trauma can be conservatively treated in 70–90% of hemodynamic stable patients, in the absence of other associated lesions/peritoneal signs or in the case of limited need for transfusions. Thus far, the main decision criteria for a surgical rather than a conservative approach to the management of liver trauma have been the hemodynamic stability and not the American Association for the Surgery of Trauma-Organ Injury Scale (AAST-OIS) grading of the lesion. Restricting the indications for a conservative treatment of liver traumas solely to the relief of hemodynamic stability seems nowadays to be unreasonable. Criteria for a conservative treatment are as follows: hemodynamic stability, limited need of blood transfusions, and non-associated visceral lesions on CT scan. In the presence of these conditions, non-operative approach can be undertaken, and the cornerstone of this treatment is transarterial angiographic embolization. Patients with complex liver trauma after stabilization should be sent to a referring, specialized center where a dedicated team is present. Nowadays, non-operative treatment is the gold standard for most of the patients with blunt liver injuries and the role of interventional radiologist is more and more determinant in the outcome of these patients.

Author details

Marco Massani*, Luca Bonariol, Bruno Pauletti, Cesare Ruffolo, Roberta Bonariol, Ezio Caratozzolo and Nicolo' Bassi

*Address all correspondence to: mmassani@ulss.tv.it

IV Department of Surgery, Center for HPB Surgery, Treviso Regional Hospital, Treviso, Italy

References

[1] Tinkoff G, Esposito TJ, Reed J, et al. American Association for the Surgery of Trauma Organ Injury Scale I: spleen, liver, and kidney, validation based on the national trauma Data Bank. J Am College of Surgeon. 2009; 207: 646–655.

[2] Richardson JD. Changes in the management of injuries to the liver and spleen. J Am Coll Surg. 2005; 200: 648–669.

[3] Joosse P, Soedarmo S, Luitse JS, Ponsen KJ. Trauma outcome analysis of a Jakarta University using the TRISS method: validation and limitation in comparison with the

major trauma outcome study. Trauma and Injury Severity Score. J Trauma. 2001; 51(1): 134–40.

[4] Baker SP, O'Neill B, Haddon W, Long WB. The injury severity score: a method for describing patients with multiple injuries and evaluating emergency care. J Trauma 1974; 14(3): 187–196.

[5] Moore EE, Cogbill TH, Jurkovich GJ, Shackford SR, Malangoni MA, Champion HR. OIS: spleen and liver (1994 revision). J Trauma 1995; 38: 323–324.

[6] Mirvis SE, Whitley NO, Vainwrigth JR, et al. Blunt hepatic trauma in adults: CT based classification and correlation with prognosis and treatment. Radiology. 1989; 171: 27–32.

[7] Karp MP, Cooney DR, Pros GA, et al. The nonoperative management of pediatric hepatic trauma. J Pediatr Surg 1983; 18: 512–518.

[8] Pachter HL, Hofstetter SR. The current status of non operative management of adult blunt hepatic injuries. Am J Surg 1995; 169: 442–454.

[9] Malhotra AK, Fabian TC, Croce MA, Gavin TJ, et al. Blunt Hepatic Injury: a paradigm shift from operative to non operative management in the 1990s. Ann Surg. 2000; 231(6): 804–813.

[10] Richardson JD, Franklin GA, Lukan JK, Carrillo EH, et al. Evolution in the management of hepatic trauma: a 25-year perspective. Ann Surg. 2000; 232(3): 324–330.

[11] Hurtuk M, Reed RL, Esposito TJ, Davis KA, Luchette FA. Trauma surgeons practice what they preach: the NTDB story on solid organ injury management. J Trauma. 2006; 61(2):243–54; discussion 254–5.

[12] Patricio MP, Brown JB, Pujana JC, et al. The swinging pendulum: a National perspective of non operative management in severe blunt liver injury. J Trauma Acute Care Surg. 2013; 75(4): 590–595.

[13] Kozar RA, Moore FA, Niles SE, et al. Complications of non operative management of high-grade blunt hepatic injuries. J Trauma. 2005; 59(5): 1066–1071.

[14] Van der Wilden GM, Velhamos GC, Emhoff T, Brancato S, Adams C, Georgakis G, Jacobs L, Gross R, Agarwal S, Burke P, et al. Successful non operative management of the most severe blunt liver incurie: a multicenter study of the research consortium of new England centers for Trauma. JAMA Surg. 2012; 147: 423–429.

[15] Bonariol L, Massani M, Caratozzolo E, Ruffolo C, et al. Management of grade III IV blunt liver traumas: a comparative, observational study. Minerva Chirurgica. 2015; 70(1): 7–15.

[16] Fang JF, Chen RJ, Wong YC, et al. Classification and treatment of pooling of contrast material in computed tomography scan of blunt hepatic injury. J Trauma. 2000; 49:1083–1088.

[17] Alarhayem AQ, Myers JG, Dent D, Lamus D, Lopera J, et al. "Blush at first sight": significance of computed tomographic and angiographic discrepancy in patients with blunt abdominal trauma. Am J Surg. 2015; 210: 1104–1111.

[18] Hagiwara A, Murata A, Matsuda T, Matsuda H. The efficacy and limitations of transarterial embolization for severe hepatic injury. J Trauma. 2002; 52(6): 1091–1096.

[19] Stassen NA, Bhullar I, Cheng JD, et al. Nonoperative management of blunt hepatic injury: an Eastern Association for the Surgery of trauma practice management guideline. J Trauma Acute Care Surg. 2012; 73(5 Suppl. 4): S288–S293.

[20] Poletti PA, Mirvis SE, Shanmuganathan K, et al. CT criteria for management of blunt liver trauma: correlation with angiographic and surgical findings. Emerg Radiol. 2000; 216(2): 418–427.

[21] Carillo E, Spain D, Wohltmann D, et al. Interventional techniques are useful adjuncts in non operative managemnet of hepatic incurie. J Trauma. 1999; 46: 619–622.

[22] Sivrikoz E, Teixeira PG, Resnick S, Inaba K, et al. Angiointervention: an independent predictor of survival in high grade blunt liver injuries. Am J Surg. 2015; 209(4): 742–746.

[23] Ward J, Alarcon L, Peitzman AB. Management of blunt liver injuries: what is new. Eur J Trauma. 2015; 41: 229–237.

[24] Mohr AM, Lavery RF, Barone A, et al. Angiographic embolization for liver injuries: low mortality, high morbidity. J Trauma. 2003; 55: 1077–1081.

[25] Letoublon C, Morra I, Chen Y, et al. Hepatic arterial embolization in the management of blunt hepatic trauma: indications and complications. J Trauma Injury Infect Crit Care. 2011; 70(5): 1032–1037.

[26] Dabbs DN, Stein DM, Scalea TM. Major hepatic necrosis: a common complication after angioembolization for treatment of high grade liver injuries. J Trauma. 2009; 66: 621–627.

[27] Kozar RA, Moore FA, Moore EE, et al. Western Trauma Association critical decision in Trauma: Non operative management of adult blunt hepatic Trauma. J Trauma Injury Infect Crit Care. 2009; 67(6): 1144–1149.

[28] Swaid F, Peleg K, Alfici R, Matter I, et al. Concomitant hollow viscus injuries in patients with blunt hepatic and splenic injuries; an analysis of a National Trauma Registry database. Injury. 2014; 45: 1409–1412.

[29] Boese CK, Hackl M, Muller P, Ruchholtz S, Michael F, Lechler P. Nonoperative management of blunt hepatic trauma: a systematic review. J Trauma Acute Care Surg. 2015; 79(4): 654–660.

[30] Fang JF, Wong YC, Lin BC, Hsu YP, Chen MF. The CT risk factors for the need of operative treatment in initially hemodynamically stable patients after blunt hepatic trauma. J Trauma. 2006; 61: 547–554.

[31] Peitzman AB, Ferrada P, Puyana JC. Nonoperative management of blunt abdominal trauma: have we gone too far. Surg Infect. 2009; 10(5): 427–433.

[32] Kozar RA, Moore FA, Cothren C, Moore EE, et al. Risk factors for hepatic morbidity following non operative management. Arch Surg. 2006; 141: 451–459.

[33] Patcher HL, Knudson MM, Ross S, Hoyt D, Cogbill T. Status of non operative management of blunt liver trauma in 1995: a multicenter experience with 404 patients. J Trauma. 1996; 40: 31–38.

[34] Carrillo EH, Wohltmann C, Richardson JD, Polk HC Jr. Evolution in the treatment of complex blunt liver injuries. Curr Probl Surg. 2001; 38: 1–60.

[35] Cox JC, Fabian TC, Maish GO 3rd, Bee TK, Pritchard FE, Russ SE, Grieger D, Winestone MI, Zarzaur BL Jr, Croce MA, et al. Routine follow-up imaging is unnecessary in the management of blunt hepatic injury. J Trauma. 2005; 59(5): 1175–1180.

[36] Pachter HL. Prometheus bound: evolution in the management of hepatic trauma – from myth to reality. Trauma Acute Care Surg. 2012; 72(2): 321–329.

[37] Piper GL, Peitzman AB. Current management of hepatic trauma. Surg Clin North Am. 2010; 90(4): 775–785.

[38] Kozar RA, Feliciano DV, Moore EE, Moore FA, Cocanour CS, West MA, Davis JW, McIntyre RC Jr. Western Trauma Association/critical decisions in trauma: operative management of adult blunt hepatic trauma. J Trauma. 2011; 71(1): 1–5.

[39] Polanco P, Leon S, Pineda J, Puyana JC, Ochoa JB, Alarcon L, Harbrecht BG, Geller D, Peitzman AB. Hepatic resection in the management of complex injury to the liver. J Trauma. 2008; 65(6): 1264–1269; discussion 1269-70. doi: 10.1097/TA.0b013e3181904749.

[40] Lin BC, Fang JF, Chen RJ, Wong YC, Hsu YP. Surgical management and outcome of blunt major liver injuries: experience of damage control laparotomy with perihepatic packing in one trauma centre. Injury. 2014; 45(1): 122–127.

[41] Li Petri S, Gruttadauria S, Pagano D, Echeverri GJ, Di Francesco F, Cintorino D, Spada M, Gridelli B. Surgical management of complex liver trauma: a single liver transplant center experience. Am Surg. 2012; 78(1): 20–25.

[42] Asensio JA, Petrone P, García-Núñez L, Kimbrell B, Kuncir E. Multidisciplinary approach for the management of complex hepatic injuries AAST-OIS grades IV-V: a prospective study. Scand J Surg. 2007; 96(3): 214–220.

[43] Peitzman AB, Marsh JW. Advanced operative techniques in the management of complex liver injury. J Trauma Acute Care Surg. 2012; 73(3): 765–770.

[44] Asensio JA, Roldán G, Petrone P, Rojo E, Tillou A, Kuncir E, Demetriades D, Velmahos G, Murray J, Shoemaker WC, Berne TV, Chan L. Operative management and outcomes in 103 AAST-OIS grades IV and V complex hepatic injuries: trauma surgeons still need to operate, but angioembolization helps. J Trauma. 2003; 54(4): 647–653.

[45] Prichayudh S, Sirinawin C, Sriussadaporn S, Pak-art R, Kritayakirana K, Samorn P, Sriussadaporn S. Management of liver injuries: predictors for the need of operation and damage control surgery. Injury. 2014; 45(9): 1373–1377.

[46] Buckman RF Jr, Miraliakbari R, Badellino MM. Juxtahepatic venous injuries: a critical review of reported management strategies. J Trauma. 2000; 48(5): 978–984.

[47] MacKenzie S, Kortbeek JB, Mulloy R, Hameed SM. Recent experiences with a multidisciplinary approach to complex hepatic trauma. Injury. 2004; 35(9): 869–877.

Chapter 10

Damage Control Surgery

Burhan Hakan Kanat, Mehmet Bugra Bozan,
Seyfi Emir, Ilhan Bali, Selim Sozen, Burak Dal and
Fatih Erol

Additional information is available at the end of the chapter

http://dx.doi.org/10.5772/64326

Abstract

Objective: The basis of damage control surgery rests on quick control of life-threatening bleeding, injuries, and septic sources in the appropriate patients before restoring their physiological reserves as a first step followed by ensuring of the physiological reserves and control of acidosis, coagulopathy, and hypothermia prior to complementary surgery.

Material and methods: Knowing when to perform damage control surgery will increase the likelihood of survival. There are three main criteria that are important in the selection of patients: (1) critical physiological factors, (2) complex injury causing the loss of physiological reserves, and (3) other conditions in trauma patients. Acidosis, acquired coagulopathy, and hypothermia (death triangle/the lethal triad) which are among critical physiological factors come to the fore in patient selection. In patients predicted to undergo damage control surgery, a replacement with crystalloids is applied after establishing a wide vascular access before reaching the hospital with the purpose of maintaining acceptable vital functions until reaching the hospital.

In the rapid/primary surgery stage, the purpose is controlling bleeding and contamination. With the purpose of controlling bleeding and hemostasis, packing, clamping, ligation, and shunting procedures are applied to the four quadrants or a balloon catheterization is done. Following hemorrhage control, the colon and intestines are examined. Primary suturation, simple resections, closed absorbent systems, and external drainage are preferred for controlling contamination. However, reconstructive surgeries, stoma forming, and nutrition ostomies are not applied in this quick laparotomy. Then, abdominal closure (temporary abdominal closures; TAC) is done. In the second stage of damage control surgery (resuscitation), patients are taken into an intensive care unit for a period of 24–48 h for the enabling of aggressive resuscitation and patient monitoring. The main objective here is the elimination of problems caused by the acidosis, coagulopathy, and hypothermia triangle. Following 24–48 h of resuscitation after primary surgery in intensive care, planned definitive surgery is performed (the third stage of damage control surgery). The packing materials are carefully removed. After all injuries are detected and any hemorrhages are stopped, complementary gastrointestinal repair (such as resections and anastomoses) is done and if it is not necessary, then ostomy and the opening of enteric feeding tubes are avoided. Closed system drainages and a nasoenteric feeding tube are placed if necessary. If abdominal closure cannot be fully done, temporary abdominal closure is done in the fourth stage.

Results: After damage control surgery procedures, there was an improvement in survival rates.

Conclusion: Damage control surgery and damage control management of the patient are important for improved survival rates and success of treatment before the lethal triad occurs deeply.

Keywords: damage control surgery, trauma, abdominal injury, sepsis, death triangle

1. Introduction

Before damage control surgery was defined, classic surgical procedures applied regardless of the physiological condition of patients would produce high rates of mortality. Prolonged intervention for definitive surgical procedures would result in the depletion of the patient's reserves and result in a process deadlier for the patients [1]. Although damage control surgery was initially planned for use on patients with severe abdominal trauma, today severely septic patients who undergo surgery are also included in this group [2, 3]. Damage control surgery continues to develop during the quarter-century period in which it was defined.

For the first time in the 1980s when the treatment principles were defined, Stone et al. stated that they reduced the high mortality rates by one-third [4]. Burch et al. [5] in an ongoing process mentioned the packing procedure in liver injury. With the start of the process, Rotondo et al. [6] mentioned "Damage Control Surgery" for the first time in 1993, and in their publication in which they applied damage control procedures to patients with major abdominal visceral and vascular injury, they stated that there was an improvement from 11 to 77% in survival rates [6].

In fact, the basis of damage control surgery rests on quick control of life-threatening bleeding, injuries, and septic sources in the appropriate patient before restoring their physiological reserves as a first step followed by ensuring of the physiological reserves and control of acidosis, coagulopathy, and hypothermia prior to complementary surgery [7]. Patients are monitored in intensive care units with the purpose of ameliorating this deadly triad and afterwards, their complementary surgeries and abdominal closing procedures are performed [1, 7].

http://dx.doi.org/10.5772/64326

2. When should damage control surgery be done?

Knowing when to perform damage control surgery will increase the likelihood of survival. There are four main topics that are important in the selection of patients: (1) critical physiological factors, (2) complex injury causing the loss of physiological reserves, and (3) other conditions in trauma patients (**Table 1**) [7].

---

1. Critical physiological factors
    - a. Hypothermia (<35°C)
    - b. Acidosis (pH < 7.2 or base deficit > 8)
    - c. Coagulopathy
        - i. Nonmechanical bleeding
        - ii. Prolonged PT
        - iii. Thrombocytopenia
        - iv. Hypofibrinemia
        - v. The need for massive transfusion (the need for more than >10 units of red blood or the need for body fluid replacement)
    - d. Prolonged time for definitive surgery (>90 minutes)
    - e. Hemodynamic instability or pre-existing hypoperfusion
2. Complex injury associated with the loss of physiological reserve
    - a. High-energy blunt trauma
    - b. Multiple penetrant injuries
    - c. Visceral injury combined with major vascular trauma
    - d. Injuries passing through body cavities (closed head trauma, major vascular injury, and pelvic trauma)
3. Other conditions in trauma patients
    - a. Injuries that are better treated by nonsurgical means such as hepatic or pelvic injury corrected with angiographic embolization
    - b. Variations in physiological reserve (the elderly, those with a large number of comorbidities, and athletes)

Table 1. Indications for patient selection for damage control surgery [7].

Acidosis, acquired coagulopathy, and hypothermia (death triangle/the lethal triad) which are among critical physiological factors come to the fore in patient selection. There is a multivariable relationship between these three basic conditions [1]. Also the hypotension that occurs emerges as an important parameter in patients on whom damage control surgery is being planned to be done.

High-energy blunt traumas that can lead to the depletion of physiological reserves, those with a large number of penetrating injuries, injuries where more than one compartment is affected, and injuries where visceral organ and vascular injuries have occurred together are indicators for damage control surgery [7].

In patients predicted to undergo damage control surgery, a replacement with crystalloids is applied after establishing a wide vascular access before reaching the hospital. The main goal of replacement therapy, especially applied to patients whose transportation to the hospital will be prolonged, is to maintain acceptable vital functions until reaching the hospital [8–10].

3. The death triangle (the lethal triad)

It consists of hypothermia, acquired coagulopathy, and acidosis and was defined for the first time by Burch et al [5]. This condition gives rise to the depletion of physiological reserves and to life-threatening consequences (**Figure 1**).

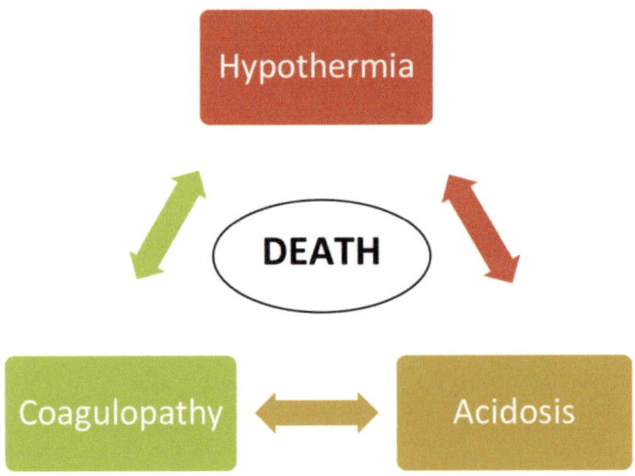

Figure 1. The death triangle (the lethal traid).

3.1. Hypothermia

Extensive injury as well as the resuscitation wherein we performed massive transfusion also contributes to its formation. Tissue hypoperfusion due to serious bleeding occurs and deterioration of oxygenation occurs as a result. Consequently, hypothermia occurs [1].

In particular, the hypothermic condition continuing below 36°C for a long time (longer than 4 h) becomes clinically significant. Mortality rates rise up to 100% in patients with multiple injuries and whose body temperature is below 32°C. The decrease in oxygenation and in tissue perfusion due to bleeding in particular plays a role in its formation [11].

If hypothermia persists, it leads to cardiac arrhythmia, decrease in cardiac output, increase in systemic vascular resistance, and a leftward shift in the oxygen dissociation curve in the long term. It also leads to the impairment of the immune system and its suppression as a result of this [12].

It also deepens acquired coagulopathy, which is another important issue (with a decrease in the activation of coagulation factors, platelet dysfunction, impairment of endothelial permeability, and stimulation of the fibrinolytic system). This results in uncontrolled bleeding.

3.2. Coagulopathy

The balance between bleeding and bleeding control mechanism is disrupted due to trauma. Although there are many underlying factors, massive transfusion and hypothermia are important.

Especially in hypothermic patients, it leads to platelet dysfunction by disrupting the interaction between von Willebrand and the platelet glycoprotein 1b-IX-V complex. A decrease in the metabolic rate of coagulation factors occurs below 35°C [13].

Massive blood transfusions lead to hemodilution and the aggravation of coagulopathy and acidosis due to this.

Although prothrombin time (PT), partial thromboplastin time (PTT), and fibrinogen levels help, clinical suspicion is essential for diagnosis. In particular, extensive hemorrhages not due to surgical causes (such as from injuries, serosal surfaces, and the skin) help in making a clinical diagnosis [1].

3.3. Metabolic acidosis

In trauma patients, anaerobic respiration increases and lactic acidosis arises due to prolonged hypoperfusion. It gets aggravated with multiple blood transfusions, aortic clamping, and insufficient myocardial functioning. As it gets aggravated, it increases coagulopathy and due to this also hypothermia [1].

4. Stages of damage control surgery

4.1. Stage I (rapid/primary surgery)

Rapid surgery is applied with the purpose of controlling bleeding and contamination. The abdomen is entered with a midline incision extending from the xiphoid to the symphysis pubis. With the purpose of controlling bleeding and hemostasis, packing, clamping, ligation, and shunting procedures are performed to the four quadrants or a balloon catheterization is done [14].

Following hemorrhage control, the colon and intestines are examined with the aim to prevent contamination. If perforation is observed, contamination is tried to be prevented by primary suturing and connecting or with a stapler. If the injured small intestine loop is below 50%, a simple single resection can be applied. Ensuring continuity of the bowel is not in the foreground. In the case of a biliary or pancreatic injury, closed absorbent systems and external drainage procedures are preferred. However, reconstructive surgeries, stoma forming, and nutrition ostomies are not applied in this quick laparotomy [1, 15].

Before the abdomen is closed, the inside of the abdomen is washed with warm solutions.

Then, abdominal closure (temporary abdominal closures; TAC) is done with the Baker technique, which today has taken the place of methods like the Bogota bag and clamping of the skin. Plastic-coated abdominal covers are laid in such a way as to protect the visceral tissues beneath and closed absorbent systems are laid on this plastic cover at the level of subcutaneous tissue. Meanwhile, the skin is protected. Ready kits are available for this technique (KCI V.A.C. and ABThera, Kinetic Concepts, Inc., San Antonio, TX; Renasys systems, Smith & Nephew, Inc., St. Petersburg, FL). In this way, the tension that causes abdominal compartment syndrome is reduced [7, 15].

In a septic abdomen, primary surgical treatment mainly focuses on controlling the contamination. To this end, resections and drainages are carried out. According to the source (hollow organ injury, pancreatic injury, or hepatobiliary injury), a wide source control can be ensured with a vacuum-aided TAC as in a trauma [7].

4.2. Stage II (resuscitation)

Following primary surgery, patients are taken into an intensive care unit for a period of 24–48 h for the enabling of aggressive resuscitation and patient monitoring. The main objective here is the elimination of problems caused by the acidosis, coagulopathy, and hypothermia triangle [1, 7, 16].

First, it is planned for the patient to be brought close to the euvolemic state to ensure end-organ perfusion. For this purpose, the patient is given blood products (such as erythrocytes and fresh frozen plasma [FFP]). The shock of the patient gets tried to be ameliorated with fluid resuscitation. Following these, techniques such as artery catheterization and pulse artery catheterization are applied [1, 17].

The hypothermic condition of the patients is important because hypothermia can cause acidosis and coagulopathy to deepen. The control of hypothermia begins with the quick termination of the initial operation. The quick removal of wet covers from the patient, raising of the room temperature in the operation room, the use of warm resuscitation fluids and ventilator air and heat regulating covers help warm up the patient in the initial surgery room. The patient should be exposed to heat for about 4 h before being taken into the intensive care unit. Pleural lavage can be applied to patients whose body temperature does not rise despite the methods applied. If the body temperature continues to be low, continuous arteriovenous heating can be applied [6, 16].

Coagulopathy is the goal as a secondary objective. For this purpose, blood products and resuscitation are planned for the patient. In the first 24 h, replacement is applied to the patient according to the rule of 10s (10 units for erythrocyte suspension, fresh frozen plasma, and platelets each) [1]. Replacement is continued until 1 PT period is 15 s and the platelet number is 100,000/mm^3. If fibrinogen levels are low, cryoprecipitate can be applied every 4 h. In life-threatening nonsurgical hemorrhages, recombinant factor VIIa can be applied [1].

If sufficient resuscitation is ensured and the patient is exposed to heat and oxygenation is ensured, then oxidative respiration increases and the acidosis is corrected by itself [17].

4.3. Stage III (definitive/complementary surgery)

Following 24–48 h of resuscitation after primary surgery in intensive care, planned definitive surgery is performed [7]. First, the packing materials of the patient are carefully removed. After which all injuries are detected and any hemorrhages are stopped. Complementary gastrointestinal repair (such as resections and anastomoses) is done and if it is not necessary, then ostomy and the opening of enteric feeding tubes are avoided. After the inside of the abdomen is cleaned, closed system drainages are placed if necessary. A nasoenteric feeding tube is placed if necessary, and if abdominal closure cannot be fully done, temporary abdominal closure is done [7]. Rapid closures, moderately rapid closures, and long-term closures are among temporary abdominal closure techniques (**Table 2**).

1.	Rapid closure	
	a.	Only skin closure
	b.	Placing a protective element such as a Bogota bag
	c.	Vacuum-aided abdominal covers
2.	Moderate closure	
	a.	Successive skin or fascial closure
	b.	Placing of interpositional mesh
	c.	Vacuum-aided abdominal covers
3.	Long-term closure (planned ventral hernia)	

Table 2. Closure options for abdominal injuries [7].

In patients with a septic abdomen, the septic source is debrided and drainage is applied. However, in order to avoid problems like abdominal compartment syndrome, relaparatomies or a planned relaparotomy can be done [7].

4.4. Stage IV (abdominal wall closure)

It is applied on patients whose abdomens could not be closed in definitive surgery and on whom temporary abdominal closure techniques are applied [15] (**Figure 2**).

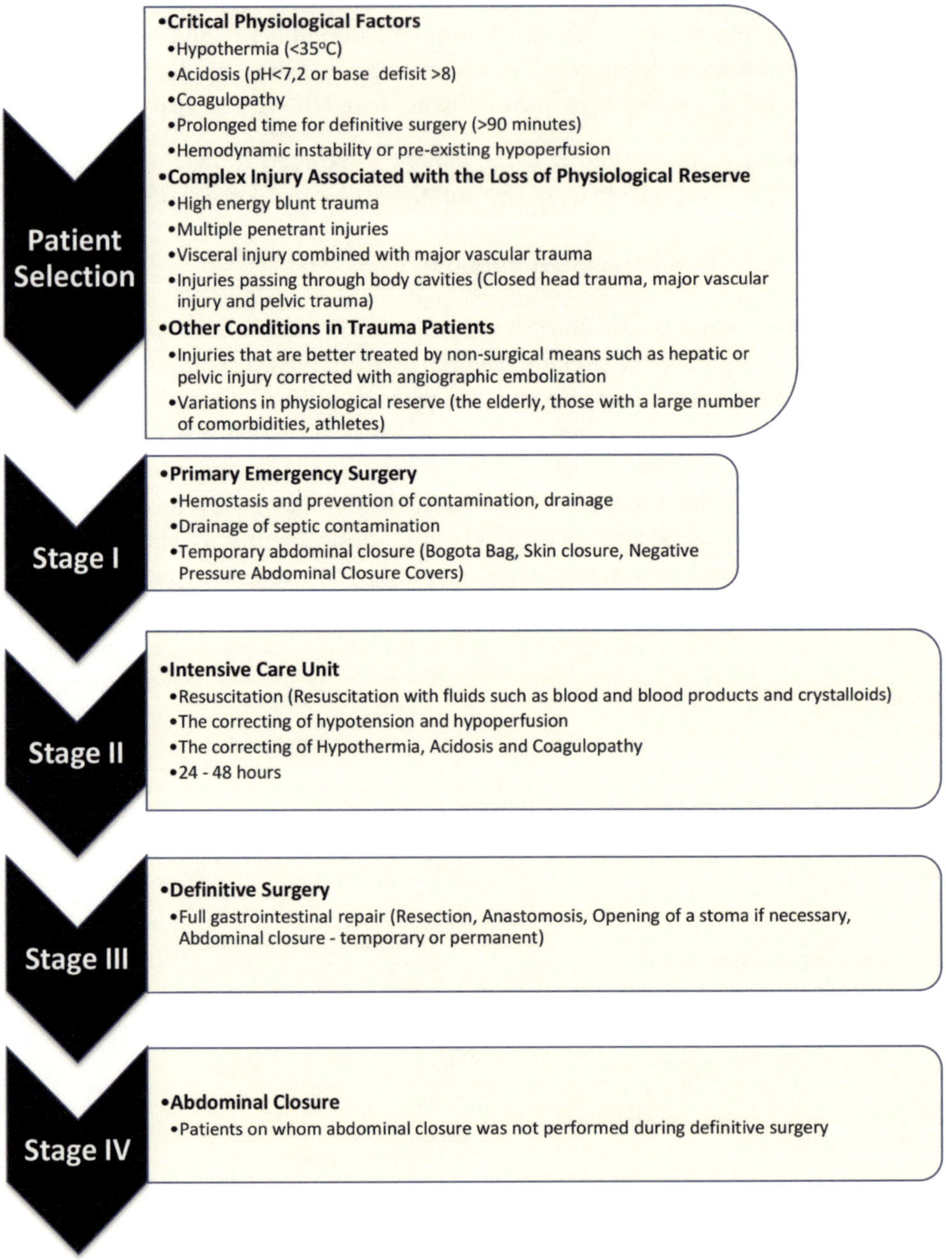

Figure 2. The stages of damage control surgery.

5. Complications

5.1. Abdominal compartment syndrome

In this condition, which arises especially after visceral swelling, hematoma, and packing procedures, a distended abdomen, increased peak airway pressure, insufficient ventilation, hypoxia, and oliguria or anuria are observed (**Table 3**) [18–20]. It can be measured with catheters placed in the bladder or catheters placed in the stomach. 35 cm H_2O is diagnostic for compartment syndrome. Rapid abdominal decompression is applied in the treatment [18].

Serious abdominal injuries
The dissolution of intestinal contents
Pressure in primary fastia closure
Abdominal packing applications for coagulation
Massive transfusion that causes intestinal edema and distension
Failures in control of hemorrhage resulting in increased acidosis and coagulopathy

Table 3. Predisposing factors for increased intra-abdominal pressure in damage control surgery [21, 22].

5.2. Enterocutaneous fistulae and wound site problems

It can be observed up to 15% in abdominal trauma patients, especially patients with sepsis. Manipulations in internal organs in particular (especially open abdomen patients with pancreatic and colonic injuries) play a role [1]. When enteroatmospheric fistulae form, it is difficult for them to close and for the wound to be protected.

Hernias are one of the most frequently encountered complications of damage control surgery because of the nature of surgical interventions with open abdomen. Intra-abdominal abscesses, surgical incisional infections, sepsis, massive blood transfusions, malnutrition, and hypoproteinemia are factors that would negatively affect the recovery of wounds and cause incisional hernia [23].

5.3. Intra-abdominal abscesses

Abscesses whose incidence increases especially with abdominal packing are observed between 10 and 70% in abdominal trauma patients. Reasons for abdominal abscesses are colonic injuries, presence of a foreign object in the abdomen for more than 24 h, inadequate drainage of seepage blood and other body fluids, and foreign objects that enter the abdomen during a penetrating injury [23, 24].

Just as it can be corrected by radiological methods, surgical drainage can also be applied.

5.4. Organ-specific complications

5.4.1. Liver

Liver-related complications (e.g., hemorrhage, hemobilia, arteriovenous fistula, pseudo-aneurysm, biloma, bile leak, and abscess formation) occur in approximately 20–45% of patients [23–25]. In diagnosis of postoperative complications such as hepatic or perihepatic abscesses or bilomas, abdominal CT and ultrasound (US) were used [23–25]. Postoperative prolonged hemorrhage can be associated with coagulopathy [25–27]. Up to 85% of majority of complications following liver trauma can be successfully managed with nonoperative techniques (such as endoscopic retrograde cholangiogram, percutaneous drainage, and angiography) [28].

5.4.2. Pancreas

Pancreatic injury is seen in 2–3% of severe abdominal injuries. Mortality due to pancreatic injury is generally caused by accompanying injuries. The most common specific complication following pancreatic injury is a pancreatic fistula (10–20%). Peripancreatic, subhepatic, and subphrenic fluid collections are commonly seen on US or CT after pancreatic trauma, and pseudocysts may occur as a result of undetected pancreatic duct disruption. Magnetic resonance cholangiopancreatography (MRCP) or endoscopic retrograde cholangiopancreatography (ERCP) provides accurate anatomical delineation of the duct injury [29].

Complications such as fistula, pseudocyst, and abscess can be treated with nonsurgical treatment by advanced radiological intervention and ERCP [29]. If this fails, operative interventions can be options for treatment of complications.

5.4.3. Colon, rectum, and small bowels

Anastomotic leakage is the most serious complication specific to intestinal surgery (2.9–15.3%) [30]. CT scan-guided percutaneous drainage should be performed in hemodynamically stable non-septic patients with a success rate of up to 80% [30].

5.5. Multiorgan failure(MOF) and acute respiratory distress syndrome (ARDS)

ARDS or MOF incidence ranges between 14 and 53%, depending on different series. In trauma patients, the risk factors of ARDS include the presence of sepsis, transfusion of more than 15 units of packed red blood cells in 24 h, pulmonary contusion, and long-bone fractures [4, 5, 31–33].

6. Conclusion

Trauma is a multisystemic and a multidisciplinary problem for physicians. Choosing the patient's appropriate treatment is the top goal of the physician. Damage control surgery and damage control management of the patient are important for improved survival rates and success of treatment before the lethal triad occurs deeply.

http://dx.doi.org/10.5772/64326

Author details

Burhan Hakan Kanat[1*], Mehmet Bugra Bozan[1], Seyfi Emir[2], Ilhan Bali[2], Selim Sozen[2], Burak Dal[3] and Fatih Erol[1]

*Address all correspondence to: burhankanat@hotmail.com

1 Training and Research Hospital, General Surgery Department, Elazığ, Turkey

2 Namik Kemal University, Faculty of Medicine, General Surgery Department, Tekirdag, Turkey

3 Iskenderun State Hospital, General Surgery Department, Hatay, Turkey

References

[1] Jaunoo SS, Harji DP. Damage Control Surgery. Int J Surg. 2009; 7: 110–113.

[2] Schecter WP, Ivatury RR, Rotondo MF, et al. Open abdomen after trauma andabdominal sepsis: a strategy for management. J Am Coll Surg. 2006; 203: 390–396.

[3] Cheatham ML, Safcsak K. Is the evolving management of intraabdominal hypertension and abdominal compartment syndrome improving survival? Crit Care Med. 2010; 38: 402–407.

[4] Stone HH, Strom PR, Mullins RJ. Management of the major coagulopathy with onset during laparotomy. Ann Surg. 1983; 197: 532–535.

[5] Burch JM, Ortiz VB, Richardson RJ, Martin RR, Mattox KL, Jordan Jr GL. Abbreviated laparotomy and planned reoperation for critically injured patients. Ann Surg. 1992; 215(5): 476–483.

[6] Rotondo MF, Schwab CW, McGonigal MD, et al. 'Damage control': an approach for improved survival in exsanguinating penetrating abdominal injury. J Trauma. 1993; 35: 375–382; discussion 382–383.

[7] Waibek BH, Rotondo MMF. Damage control surgery: it's evolution over the last 20 years. Rev Col Bras Cir. 2012; 39: 314–321.

[8] Soreide E, Deakin CD. Pre-hospital fluid therapy in the critically injured patient—a clinical update. Injury. 2005; 36: 1001–1010.

[9] Rhee P, Koustova E, Alam HB. Searching for the optimal resuscitation method: recommendations for the initial fluid resuscitation of combat casualties. J Trauma. 2003; 54: 52–62.

[10] Dawes R, Thomas GO. Battlefield resuscitation. Curr Opin Crit Care. 2009; 15: 527–535.

[11] Jurkovich G, Greiser W, Luterman A, Curreri PW. Hypothermia in trauma victim: an ominous predictor of survival. J Trauma. 1987; 27: 1019–1024.

[12] Cosgriff N, Moore FE, Sauaia A, Kenny-Moynihan M, Burch JM, Galloway B. Predicting life-threatening coagulopathy in the massively transfused trauma patient: hypothermia and acidosis revisited. J Trauma. 1997; 42: 857–862.

[13] Kermode JC, Zheng Q, Milner EP. Marked temperature dependence of the platelet calcium signal induced by human von Willebrand factor. Blood. 1999; 94: 199–207.

[14] Germanos S, Gourgiotis S, Villias C, Bertucci M, Dimopoulos N, Salemis N. Damage control surgery in the abdomen: An approach for the management of severe injured patients. Int J Surg. 2008; 6: 246–252.

[15] Miller PR, Thompson JT, Faler BJ, et al. Late fascial closure in lieu of ventral hernia: the next step in open abdomen management. J Trauma. 2002; 53: 843–849.

[16] Asensio JA, McDuffie L, Petrone P, Roldan G, Forno W, Gambaro E, et al. Reliable variables in the exsanguinated patient which indicate damage control and predict outcome. Am J Surg. 2001; 182: 743–751.

[17] Parr MJA, Alabdi T. Damage control surgery and intensive care. Injury. 2004; 35: 713–722.

[18] Burch JM, Moore EE, Moore FA, Francoise R. The abdominal compartment syndrome. Surg Clin North Am. 1996; 76: 833–839.

[19] Meldrum DR, Moore FA, Moore EE, Francoise RJ, Sauaia A, Burch JM. Prospective characterisation and selective management of the abdominal compartment syndrome. Am J Surg. 1997; 174: 667–672.

[20] Morris JA, Eddy VA, Blinman TA, Rutherford EF, Sharp KW. The staged celiotomy for trauma: issues in unpacking and reconstruction. Ann Surg. 1993; 217: 576–584.

[21] Gentilello LM, Pierson DJ. Trauma critical care. Am J Respir Crit Care Med. 2001; 163: 604–607.

[22] Kouraklis G, Spirakos S, Glivanou A. Damage control surgery: an alternative approach for the management of critically injured patients. Surg Today. 2002; 32: 195–202.

[23] Simsek A, Ozer MT, Eryilmaz M, Ozturk E, Ozerhan IH, Gorgulu S, Peker Y, Tufan CT. The results of damage control surgery in abdominal trauma. Balk Mil Med Rev. 2007; 10(3): 136–140.

[24] Shapiro MB, Jenkins DH, Schwab W, et al. Damagecontrol collective review. J Trauma. 2000; 49: 969–978.

[25] Doklestić K, Stefanović B, Gregorić P, Ivančević N, Lončar Z, Jovanović B, Bumbaširević V, Jeremić V, Vujadinović ST, Stefanović B, Milić N, Karamarković A. Surgical management of AAST grades III-V hepatic trauma by damage control surgery with

perihepatic packing and definitive hepatic repair–single centre experience. World J Emerg Surg. 2015; 10: 34. DOI: 10.1186/s13017-015-0031-8

[26] Piper GL, Peitzman AB. Current management of hepatic trauma. Surg Clin North Am. 2010;90:775–785.

[27] Bala M, Gazalla SA, Faroja M, Bloom AI, Zamir G, Rivkind AI, et al. Complications of high grade liver injuries: management and outcomewithfocus on bile leaks. Scand J Trauma Resusc Emerg Med. 2012; 20: 20.

[28] Howdieshell TR, Purvis J, Bates WB, Teeslink CR. Biloma and biliary fistula following hepatorraphy for liver trauma: incidence, natural history, and management. Am Surg. 1995; 61: 165–168.

[29] Krıgel JEJ, Benıngfıeld SJ, Nıcol AJ, Navsarıa P. The management of complex pancreatic İnjuries. Sajs. 2005; 43(3): 92–102.

[30] Kirchhoff P, Clavien PA, Hahnloser D. Complications in colorectal surgery: risk factors and preventive strategies. Patient Safety Surg. 2010; 4: 5. doi:10.1186/1754-9493-4-5

[31] Schreiber MA. Dmage Control Surgery. Crit Care Clin. 2004; 20 (1); 101 –118.

[32] Offner PJ, de Souza AL, Moore EE, et al. Avoidance of abdominal compartment syndrome in damage-control laparotomy after trauma. Arch Surg. 2001; 136: 676–681.

[33] Hudson LD, Milberg JA, Anardi D, et al. Clinical risks for development of the acute respiratory distress syndrome. Am J Respir Crit Care Med. 1995; 151: 293–301.

Section 3

Pediatric Surgery

Chapter 11

Emergency Abdominal Surgery in Infants and Children

Mehrdad Hosseinpour and Bahareh Ahmadi

Additional information is available at the end of the chapter

http://dx.doi.org/10.5772/63649

Abstract

The term acute abdomen refers to sudden severe abdominal pain with unclear etiology that is less than 24 h in duration. In children, acute abdominal pain presents a diagnostic dilemma. Although many cases of acute abdominal pain are benign, some of them need rapid diagnosis and treatment to minimize morbidity. The present chapter provides an overview of abdominal surgical emergencies in children and discusses the most common disorders that cause surgical acute abdomen.

Keywords: acute abdomen, infants, children, surgery, neonates

1. Introduction

1.1. Acute abdomen

The term acute abdomen refers to sudden severe abdominal pain with unclear etiology that is less than 24 h in duration. In many cases, there is a medical emergency that requires urgent and specific diagnosis. The causes of these emergencies include inflammation, abdominal organ ischemia, obstruction, hollow organ perforation, and gastrointestinal bleeding.

In children, acute abdominal pain presents a diagnostic dilemma. Although many cases of acute abdominal pain are benign, some of them require rapid diagnosis and treatment to minimize morbidity.

The most common nonsurgical condition is gastroenteritis, whereas the most common surgical condition is appendicitis. Abdominal pain in children varies with age, associated symptoms, and pain location. Meticulous history and physical examinations are essential to determine the cause of acute abdominal pain and to identify the surgical conditions, such as appendicitis.

1.2. Evaluation of the acute abdomen in children

The most appropriate therapy should then be initiated when the child's clinical status optimized. The workup should first include a thorough but efficient acquisition of the child's history and physical examination followed by the judicious use of laboratory and radiologic studies. The evaluation of children with acute abdominal pain can pose a diagnostic challenge on physicians as children may present with atypical symptoms that interfere with the usual Pattern of recognition that often guide decision making. Children are often unable to provide the desired information, which makes recognition of the cause of abdominal complaints more difficult.

Appendicitis
Meckel`s diverticulum
Intussusceptions
Intestinal malrotation
Midgut volvulus
Adhesive bowel obstruction
Testicular/ovarian torsion
Incarcerated inguinal hernia
Omental torsion
Cholecystitis
Pancreatitis
Intra-abdominal malignancies
Abdominal trauma
Surgical causes of constipation

Table 1. The most common surgical causes of acute abdomen in children.

Birth to 1 year	2 to 5 years	6 to 11 years
Intussusception	Appendicitis	Appendicitis
Hirshsprung`s disease	Incarcerated hernia	Cholecystitis
Incarcerated hernia	Intussusception	Pancreatitis
Volvulus	Volvulus	Testicular/ovarian torsion
	Trauma	Trauma
	Meckel`s diverticulum	

Table 2. Differential diagnosis of surgical acute abdomen by predominant age.

http://dx.doi.org/10.5772/63649

The present chapter provides an overview of abdominal surgical emergencies in children and discusses the most common disorders that cause surgical acute abdomen (**Table 1**). **Table 2** shows the differential diagnosis of surgical acute abdomen by predominant age.

2. Main body

2.1. Surgical acute abdomen in neonates

2.1.1. Gastric volvulus

Gastric volvulus is a rare, potentially life-threatening condition [1]. It may be defined as an abnormal rotation of one part of the stomach around another; the degree of the torsion varies from 180° to 360° and is associated with closed-loop obstruction and the risk of strangulation.

2.1.1.1. Clinical features

Clinical features depend on the degree of rotation and obstruction. Persistent regurgitation and vomiting (sometimes unproductive) are common. The vomiting may or may not contain bile, depending on pyloric obstruction. Hematemesis and anemia are well described in this disease.

2.1.1.2. Diagnosis

Plain abdominal pain and chest X-rays are essential. A distended stomach in an abnormal position should suggest the possibility of gastric volvulus.

Contrast studies clarify the anatomy and the site of obstruction, which is usually at the pylorus, giving a so-called "beak" deformity.

2.1.1.3. Treatment

Acute gastric volvulus requires appropriate resuscitation and urgent surgery if ischemic necrosis and gastric perforation are to be avoided.

If possible, the stomach should be decompressed preoperatively by nasogastric suction but vigorous attempts to pass a tube must be avoided because of a risk of gastric perforation.

2.1.2. Gastric perforation

Gastric perforation in neonates can be broadly categorized as spontaneous (idiopathic), ischemic, and traumatic; however, in many instances, the etiology may be multifactorial [2].

Neonatal gastric perforation can occur in full-term, premature, and small gestational age neonates.

Traumatic perforation results from pneumatic distention during mask ventilation, positive-pressure ventilation, or iatrogenic injury during gastric intubation.

2.1.2.1. Clinical features

The majority cases present within the first 7 days of life. The neonates are often premature or have a history of asphyxia or hypoxia. They may present with feeding intolerance or emesis (sometimes bloody). Many develop abrupt onset of rapidly progressive abdominal distention.

The abdomen may rapidly become tense and tender with signs of peritonitis. Subcutaneous emphysema in the abdominal wall or pneumoscrotum may be perceived.

2.1.2.2. Diagnosis

In infants with massive pneumoperitoneum, a plain abdominal X-ray will demonstrate air under the diaphragm. Other plain X-ray findings include subcutaneous emphysema, ascites, pneumoscrotum, or an oro-nasogastric tube outside the confines of the stomach.

2.1.2.3. Treatment

Open exploration (or laparoscopic) and repair is the essential part of treatment. However, infants with gastric perforation develop septic parameters and need to be well resuscitated preoperatively (respiratory supports, hydration, and broad spectrum antibiotics).

2.1.3. Duodenal obstruction

Congenital duodenal obstruction is the most common cause of intestinal obstruction in the newborn period [3].

Duodenal obstruction is the result of intrinsic lesions (atresia, stenosis, and "windsock" web), extrinsic lesions (annular pancreas, malrotation, preduodenal portal vein), or a combination of both.

2.1.3.1. Clinical features

About half of these patients are premature and have low birth weight. Vomiting is the most common symptom and is usually presented in the first day of life. There is minimal or no abdominal distension. The neonate may pass some meconium in the first 24 h of life.

2.1.3.2. Diagnosis

The diagnosis of duodenal obstruction is confirmed on X-ray examination. An abdominal X-ray will show a dilated stomach and duodenum (double-bubble sign), with no gas beyond the duodenum. In partial obstruction, there is usually some air in the distal intestine.

In some cases of partial duodenal obstruction, plain films may be normal. Upper gastrointestinal tract contrast X-ray is indicated in these patients to establish the diagnosis.

2.1.3.3. Treatment

Although duodenal atresia is a relative emergency, the patient should be hemodynamically stable preoperatively. Duodenoduodenostomy is the preferred procedure for patients with duodenal atresia.

2.1.4. Malrotation and midgut volvulus

Malrotation is the term used to denote an interference with normal process of orderly return of the fetal intestine from the physiological hernia to the abdominal cavity during which it undergoes systematic rotation and fixation [4].

2.1.4.1. Clinical features

Fifty-five percent of malrotations present within the first week of life and 80% in the first month. Recurrent episodes of subacute obstruction with intermittent bilious vomiting are the main symptoms in neonatal period.

Strangulating intestinal obstruction as a consequence of midgut volvulus can present as bile-stained vomiting, which may contain altered blood, abdominal distension and tenderness, the passage of dark blood per rectum, and shock. As the strangulation progresses to gangrene, perforation and peritonitis become evident.

2.1.4.2. Diagnosis

The plain abdominal X-ray in the infant with midgut volvulus typically shows a "gasless" appearance with air in the stomach and duodenum. Contrast studies are diagnostic (upper gastrointestinal contrast study). It shows the abnormal configuration of duodenum, (deviation of duodenojejunal junction to the right of midline). When volvulus has occurred, the duodenum and jejunum show a "corkscrew" appearance.

Ultrasonography to determine the relationship between the superior mesenteric vein (SMV) and the superior mesenteric artery (SMA) has been advocated.

2.1.4.3. Treatment

The operative correction of a malrotation should be regarded as a surgical emergency. Neonates presenting with acute strangulating obstruction as a result of midgut volvulus require a short period of intensive resuscitation preoperatively.

The volvulus occurs around the base of the narrowed midgut mesentery. The twist occurs in a clockwise direction and is untwisted by counter-clockwise rotation. In patients with extensive intestinal gangrene, frankly necrotic bowel should be resected and the bowel ends either tide off or stomas fashioned with a view to a second-look laparotomy in 24–48 h later.

In uncomplicated malrotation, Ladd's procedure (division of extensions of peritoneal folds across the bowel) is the preferred treatment.

2.1.5. Jejuno-ileal atresia

Jejuno-ileal atresia, defined as a congenital defect in continuity of the bowel, is a common cause of intestinal obstruction in the newborn [5].

2.1.5.1. Clinical features

Jejunoileal atresia presents clinically as neonatal intestinal obstruction with persistent bile-stained vomiting. Abdominal distension is frequently present. Constipation is usually not absolute and the meconium passed.

2.1.5.2. Diagnosis

Plain abdominal X-ray will reveal distended small bowel loops and air-fluid levels. When the abdominal X-ray suggests a complete obstruction, a contrast enema may be performed to exclude colonic atresia. The classical appearance of the colon distal to jejunoileal atresia is an-used or microcolon.

2.1.5.3. Treatment

The operation should not be delayed unduly as there is always a danger of further infarction of the bowel. The main surgical treatment in jejunoileal atresia is resection and anastomosis of bowel ends.

2.1.6. Meconium ileus

Meconium ileus is an early manifestation of cystic fibrosis (CF) due to abnormal, inspissated, and viscid mucus of intestinal origin. In children, the impacted meconium produces an intraluminal obstruction occurring in the mid-ileum, leading to a progressive abdominal distention, intestinal volvulus, atresia, gangrene, perforation, peritonitis with abdominal calcifications, and meconial pseudocyst [6].

2.1.6.1. Clinical features

A family history of cystic fibrosis is clearly evident in 25% of patients. Main symptoms include abdominal distension, bilious vomiting, and delayed passage of meconium. Meconium ileus can be recognized clinically as two different conditions: a simple, uncomplicated type not requiring surgery and a complicated, severe type.

In the first type, symptoms of a distal ileal obstruction are seen not later than 48 h after birth. These generalized abdominal distention, bilious vomiting, and no stool.

In the second type, the progressive abdominal distension may culminate in respiratory distress. If a perforation occurs, a pneumoperitoneum and sepsis will be the unfavorable consequences.

Sometimes, the onset is directly with meconium peritonitis, which could involute in a giant meconial pseudocyst.

2.1.6.2. Diagnosis

A water-soluble contrast enema is useful for both diagnosis and therapeutic purposes. Contrast enema shows microcolon appearance and pellets in terminal ileum.

2.1.6.3. Treatment

The first step of treatment includes medical management, such as nasogastric tube decompression, antibiotics, correction of dehydration, and contrast enema with water-soluble contrasts (Gastrografin, Golytely, N-Acetylcysteine).

When medical treatment is unsuccessful in spite of an uncomplicated meconium ileus, surgery is mandatory, and an open evacuation, resection, and ileostomy are the possible options.

The indication of operation for newborns with meconium peritonitis is a clear sign of intestinal obstruction or perforation. Infants with neonatal meconium calcifications, meconium ascites with hydrocele, or calcified meconium found in the hernia sac do not require operation.

2.1.7. Necrotizing enterocolitis (NEC)

NEC is the most common medical and surgical emergency affecting the gastrointestinal tract of infants in the neonatal intensive-care unit (NICU) [7]. Multiple risk factors that have been implicated in the pathogenesis of NEC include prematurity, hypoxia, initiation of enteral feeding, congenital heart disease, and bacterial infection. The majority of cases develop in infants less than 36 weeks of gestational age.

NEC is characterized by intestinal inflammation and mucosal destruction. In its most severe form, NEC is characterized by full-thickness necrosis, intestinal perforation, peritonitis, sepsis, and death.

Grade 1	Mild systemic signs (apnea, bradycardia, and temperature instability)
	Mild intestinal signs (abdominal distension, gastric residual, And occult blood in stool)
Grade 2	Mild-to-moderate systemic signs
	Additional intestinal signs (absent bowel sounds, abdominal tenderness)
	Radiologic signs (pneumatosis intestinal, portal venous air)
	Laboratory changes (metabolic acidosis, thrombocytopenia)
Grade 3	Severe systemic illness (hypotension, shock)
	Intestinal signs (large abdominal distension, abdominal wall discoloration, peritonitis, perforation)
	Severe radiologic signs (ascites, pneumoperitoneum)
	Progressive laboratory derangement (metabolic acidosis, DIC)

Table 3. Modified Bell`s stage.

2.1.7.1. Clinical features

NEC may present as feeding intolerance, abdominal distension, bloody stool, hypoxia, and shock. The bell criteria (**Table 3**) allow for categorization of the severity of NEC for treatment guidelines.

Laboratory abnormalities in NEC include thrombocytopenia, leukocytosis or leukopenia, metabolic acidosis, hypercapnea, and hypoxia.

2.2. Surgical acute abdomen in children

2.2.1. Appendicitis

Appendicitis is a common cause of emergency abdominal surgery in children [8]. Variability in clinical findings often leads to misdiagnosis.

2.2.1.1. Clinical features

Interpretation of signs requires a great deal of clinical experience of examination. History and physical examination alone show a diagnostic accuracy of approximately 90%. Acute appendicitis in children is diagnosed mainly on the basis of classical symptoms of migratory right iliac fossa pain, nausea and vomiting, right-lower quadrant (RLQ) tenderness with rebound phenomenon.

In most cases, pain is initially located periumblically and subsequently shifts to the RLQ. Fever is often present. The examiner should always consider possible atypical clinical presentation. Another important point to remember is perforation followed by a calm period (closed-cavity theory) in which pain subsides until signs of peritonitis appear.

2.2.1.2. Diagnosis

Laboratory tests including white blood cell (WBC) count and C-reactive protein (CRP) measurement do not provide additional information in the diagnosis of appendicitis.

Abdominal ultrasonography is an excellent screening tool for acute appendicitis. Computerized tomography (CT) scan has a slightly higher sensitivity and specificity than ultrasonography, and is associated with a lower negative appendectomy.

2.2.1.3. Treatment

The generally accepted treatment for appendicitis is appendectomy. Although it has been suggested that nonoperative treatment of children with uncomplicated appendicitis may be successful, there is no adequate evidence to advocate this method.

The treatment of appendicitis begins with intravenous fluid and broad-spectrum antibiotics. Management often initiating antimicrobial theory depends on the severity of inflammation (uncomplicated or non-perforated versus complicated or perforated appendicitis).

http://dx.doi.org/10.5772/63649

The current standard of care for uncomplicated appendicitis is appendectomy (open or laparoscopic). The management of complicated appendicitis can be separated into nonoperative and operative treatment.

The concept of complicated appendicitis management with antibiotics alone is to decrease the significant local and regional inflammation. Once treated, most surgeons will perform interval appendectomy often 6–10 weeks later. The majority of patients who present with a well-formed abscess on initial imaging are managed nonoperatively. Primary treatment of the abscess with antibiotics alone, or antibiotics and percutaneous drainage is a widely accepted treatment strategy. Interval appendectomy is then performed after the inflammation has subsided.

2.2.2. Intussusception

Intussusception is the most frequent cause of bowel obstruction in infants and toddlers [9]. It is acquired invagination of the proximal bowel into the distal bowel, causing obstruction of the mesenteric vessels, and eventually ischemia and necrosis of bowel. There may or may not be a lead point. The vast majorities of cases do not have a lead point and are classified as primary or idiopathic. The most common lead point is a Meckel diverticulum followed by polyps and duplication.

2.2.2.1. Clinical features

The classic presentation is an infant or a young child with intermittent, crampy abdominal pain associated with "currant jelly" stool and a palpable mass on physical examination, although this triad is seen in less than a fourth of children. The abdominal pain is sudden and the child may stiffen and pull the legs up to the abdomen. Between pain attacks, the child may appear comfortable but eventually will become lethargic. Physical examination is relatively nonspecific. There may be an abdominal mass, abdominal tenderness, and distension. Prolapse of the intussusception through the anus is a grave sign.

2.2.2.2. Diagnosis

Plain flat and upright abdominal radiography have a low accuracy for the diagnosis of intussusception, and are not used as the sole diagnostic test. X-ray can be useful in identifying free air, and indicating perforation. Ultrasound imaging is the preferred method to diagnosis intussusception. The characteristic finding on ultrasound has been referred to as a "target" or a "doughnut" lesion, which consists of alternating rings of low and high echogenicity representing the bowel wall and mesenteric for within the intussusception in a transverse plan. The pseudo kidney's sign is seen on longitudinal section. Contrast enema is also accurate, but is invasive and requires radiation.

2.2.2.3. Treatment

An air or a contrast enema is the first-line treatment as long as there are no contraindications to nonoperative management. Evidence of shock, peritonitis, sepsis, or perforation is the contraindication of enema reduction.

Surgery (open or laparoscopic) is necessary if enema reduction fails or is contraindicated.

2.2.3. *Meckel diverticulum*

Meckel diverticulum is a remnant of the embryologic vitelline (omphalomesenteric) duct that connects the fetal gut with the yolk sac and normally involutes between the fifth and seventh weeks of gestation [10]. Failure of duct regression results in a variety of abnormalities arising from persistence of the remnant. The most common anomaly (90%) is the classic Meckel diverticulum.

2.2.3.1. *Clinical features*

Gastrointestinal manifestations of Meckel diverticulum include in order of frequency, bleeding, intestinal obstruction, And inflammation of the diverticulum.

Episodic painless rectal bleeding in a young child is the classic presentation of a bleeding Meckel diverticulum. It results from ulceration of heterotopic acid-producing gastric mucosa of diverticulum.

Bowel obstruction is usually caused by a forbidden band between the umbilical and Meckel diverticulum.

Inflammation of the diverticulum (diverticulitis) is often attributed to the presence of heterotopic gastric or pancreatic tissue and is often misdiagnosed as appendicitis owing to its similar clinical course.

2.2.3.2. *Diagnosis*

In children presenting with obstruction or inflammation, the diagnosis of a Meckel diverticulum is not typically determined preoperatively. Meckel diverticulitis should be ruled out in any patient with a negative appendectomy. Technetium scan is commonly used to demonstrate heterotopic acid-producing mucosa of Meckel diverticulum.

2.2.3.3. *Treatment*

The treatment for symptomatic Meckel diverticulum consists of resection using either an open or a laparoscopic approach. Resection may be accomplished by either simple diverticulectomy or segmental ileal resection with anastomosis.

2.2.4. *Inguinal hernia*

Inguinal hernia is one of the most common surgical diseases [11]. Approximately 1–5% of all children will develop an inguinal hernia and a positive family history is found in about 10%. The incidence of an inguinal hernia varies directly with the degree of prematurity.

2.2.4.1. *Clinical features*

Most hernias are asymptomatic for inguinal bulging with straining. They are often found by the parents or pediatrician on routine physical examination. Most hernias reduce without treatment or can be reduced easily with a little manual pressure.

Incarcerated inguinal hernia is an emergency. The incidence of hernia incarceration is variable and ranges from 12 to 17%. Symptoms of incarceration are frequently manifested as a fussy or inconsolable infant with intermittent abdominal pain and vomiting. A tender and sometimes erythematic irreducible mass is noted in the groin. Abdominal distension and bloody stool are late signs. Prolonged incarceration may be associated with signs of intestinal obstruction, including poor feeding and vomiting.

2.2.4.2. *Diagnosis*

Inguinal hernia is a clinical diagnosis. If there are doubts about diagnosis, ultrasonography can confirm the diagnosis before the operation.

2.2.4.3. *Treatment*

Inguinal hernias that are easily reduced can be operated on electively (open or laparoscopic). An incarcerated hernia requires urgent reduction with firm and continuous manual pressure on the hernia mass. The presence of peritonitis or septic shock is an absolute contraindication to attempted reduction. Symptoms of bowel obstruction are a relative contraindication. Successful reduction is usually confirmed by a sudden "POP" of the contents back into the peritoneal cavity. Urgent operation is necessary if reduction fails.

2.2.5. *Trauma*

Trauma is the leading cause of morbidity and mortality in children from age 1 to 14 years [12]. Approximately 10% of pediatric hospitalizations and 15% of pediatric intensive care unit (PICU) admissions dedicates to traumas. Serious intra-abdominal injuries occur in 8% of pediatric trauma victims and are caused by crushing the solid upper abdominal viscera against the vertebral column. Injuries to the liver (27%), spleen (27%), kidneys (25%), and gastrointestinal tract (21%) occur most frequently.

2.2.5.1. *Clinical features*

While the examination can be challenging given the development level of the child, the use of comfort strategies and distraction can calm the child. Important physical findings include vital signs, abdominal contusions or abrasions, tenderness, or distension. Particular physical findings such as the seat-belt sign are suspicious for the presence of intra-abdominal injury.

2.2.5.2. *Diagnosis*

Sonography has an adjunctive role in the imaging of pediatric abdominal trauma. Focused abdominal sonography for trauma (FAST) itself is most useful in detecting intra- abdominal blood, but is not sufficiently reliable to exclude blunt abdominal injuries.

CT of abdomen should be obtained in intubated patients, patients with internal bleeding (abdominal tenderness, distension, bruising, or gross hematuria), and evidence of femur fracture, elevation of serum transaminase levels, significant microscopic hematuria, and in severe injuries.

2.2.5.3. Treatment

Most of the abdominal injuries in children can be managed nonoperatively.

2.2.5.4. Indication of emergent laparotomy:

The indication of emergent laparotomy is as follows:

1. Evidence of ongoing bleeding with an abnormal abdominal examination or a positive abdominal FAST examination.

2. Signs of peritoneal irritation.

3. Pneumoperitoneum.

4. Intraperitoneal ruptures of the urinary bladder.

5. Penetrating renal injury, however, selective observation is also being applied.

6. Hemodynamic instability regardless of resuscitation.

7. Diaphragmatic injury: emergent operative exploration in these patients is indicated in the hemodynamically unstable patients with multiple organ injuries.

3. Conclusion

An expeditious workup is necessary when evaluating children presenting with acute abdominal pain to determine the most likely cause of their symptoms and determine whether or not emergent operative intervention is necessary.

Author details

Mehrdad Hosseinpour* and Bahareh Ahmadi

*Address all correspondence to: meh_hosseinpour@yahoo.com

Imam Hossein Children Hospital, Isfahan University of Medical Sciences, Isfahan, Iran

References

[1] Porcaro F, Mattioli G, Romano C. Pediatric gastric volvulus: diagnostic and clinical approach. Case Rep Gastroenterol. 2013;7:63–8. DOI:10.1159/000348758.

[2] Lin CM, Lee HC, Kao HA, Hung HY, Hsu CH, Yeung CY, Sheu JC, Wang NL. Neonatal gastric perforation: report of 15 cases and review of the literature. Pediatr Neonatol. 2008;49(3): 65–70. DOI: 10.1016/S1875-9572(08)60015-7.

[3] Escobar MA, Ladd AP, Grosfeld JL, West KW, Rescorla FJ, Scherer LR 3rd, Engum SA, Rouse TM, Billmire DF. Duodenal atresia and stenosis: long-term follow-up over 30 years. J Pediatr Surg. 2004; 39(6):867–71. DOI:10.1016/j.jpedsurg.2004.02.025.

[4] Millar AJ, Rode H, Cywes S. Malrotation and volvulus in infancy and childhood. Semin Pediatr Surg. 2003;12(4):229–36. DOI:10.1053/j.sempedsurg.2003.08.003.

[5] Touloukian RJ. Diagnosis and treatment of jejunoileal atresia.World J Surg. 1993;17(3): 310–7.

[6] Gorter RR, Karimi A, Sleeboom C, Kneepkens CM, Heij HA. Clinical and genetic characteristics of meconium ileus in newborns with and without cystic fibrosis. J Pediatr Gastroenterol Nutr. 2010;50(5):569–72. DOI: 10.1097/MPG.0b013e3181bb3427.

[7] Thompson AM, Bizzarro MJ. Necrotizing enterocolitis in newborns: pathogenesis, prevention and management. Drugs. 2008;68(9):1227–38.

[8] Leung A, Sigalet D. Acute abdominal pain in children. Am Fam Physician. 2003; 67(11): 2321–7.

[9] Kaiser AD, Applegate KE, Ladd AP. Current success in the treatment of intussusception in children. Surgery. 2007;142(4):469–75. DOI:10.1016/j.surg.2007.07.015.

[10] Jayesh Sagar, Vikas Kumar, and DK Shah. Meckel's diverticulum: a systematic review. J R Soc Med. 2006; 99(10): 501–5. DOI: 10.1258/jrsm.99.10.501.

[11] Hardy A, Butler B, Crandall M. The evaluation of the acute abdomen. In: Moore LJ, Turner KL, Todd SR, editors. Common problems in acute care surgery: Springer; New York; 2013. p. 19–30. DOI: 10.1007/978-1-4614-6123-4-1.

[12] McFadyen JG, Ramaiah R, Bhananker SM. Initial assessment and management of pediatric trauma patients. Int J Crit Illn Inj Sci. 2012; 2(3): 121–7. DOI: 10.4103/2229-5151.100888.

Chapter 12

Anesthetic Management of Neonatal Emergency Abdominal Surgery

Esra Caliskan

Additional information is available at the end of the chapter

http://dx.doi.org/10.5772/63567

Abstract

Anesthetic management of neonatal surgical emergencies presents serious difficulties and challenges for the anesthesiologist and is associated with increased risks of morbidity and mortality. Therefore, in these patients, anesthetic assessment should be directed to the patient's current disease and associated anomalies. The provision of safe anesthesia and perioperative management of these cases also depends on a clear understanding of the physiologic and hemodynamic variables of the preterm and term infants and a precise knowledge of the pathophysiology of disease states likely to affect the neonate. This chapter describes physiology and pathophysiology-based view on the neonatal abdominal emergency surgeries. General principles of surgery and anesthetic management of specific neonatal emergencies that include congenital diaphragmatic hernia (CDH), abdominal wall defects, necrotizing enterocolitis, and esophageal atresia are reviewed and discussed.

Keywords: neonatal, emergency abdominal surgery, pediatric anesthesia, neonatal physiology, perioperative anesthetic management

1. Introduction

Advances in obstetrics and neonatology have greatly improved neonatal survival especially for infants with complex anatomical defect and preterm neonates. Most of these anotomical abnormalities to be corrected by surgical interventions after birth, some of them also corrected by intervention before birth [1, 2]. Advances in prenatal diagnosis and survival rate in these patients have resulted in an increase in the anesthetic and surgical approach. Emergency surgical conditions can be life threatening in the neonatal period. Therefore, anesthesiologists must know and better understand the distinctive physiological characteristics of neonates than of adults so that they can have information about response to anesthesia and surgery.

The purpose of this chapter is to provide basic information that will help anesthesiologists to better approach the problems of neonates. The present considerations recommend that to provide safe care these patients are also reviewed.

In this context, anesthetic management will be presented in selected neonatal surgical emergencies including congenital diaphragmatic hernia (CDH), abdominal wall defect (gastroschisis and omphalocele) necrotizing enterocolitis, and esophageal atresia. Clinical presentation and associated anomalies, perioperative approach, surgical stabilization, and postoperative follow-up period are explained and discussed.

2. Physiological features in neonates

2.1. Respiratory system

Lung development can be divided into five stages [3]. In literature and textbook knowledge reviewed, the last stage begins at about 36 weeks' gestation and continues until at least 18 months [4]. Tip II pneumocytes are responsible for surfactant production. These begin to differentiate at 24 weeks' gestation, but surfactant level is not adequate to ensure appropriate pulmonary function until 34–36 weeks of gestation [4, 3]. Therefore, respiratory immaturity and potential for respiratory distress are well-defined entities in the preterm neonate due to a deficiency of surfactant.

One of the characteristics of the fetal circulation is high pulmonary vascular resistance (PVR) [3]. PVR reduces by approximately 10% after labor, but the apparent decrease occurs with the first breath [5]. Pulmonary blood flow and alveolar and arterial PO_2 increase along with the expansion of the lung [5]. These changes are important for modification of the fetal circulation to the adult form of circulation [3, 6]. Over the next 1–2 months, PVR decreases to adult levels.

The differences in the neonatal respiratory system from that of the adult can be summarized as follows:

- Central control of ventilation is not fully developed.
- Response to hypoxia is immature.
- Peripheral feedback mechanisms are not sufficiently mature.
- Neonatal oxygen consumption per kilogram of body weight is twice as much as an adult.
- Lower functional residual capacity (moderate decrease in value of inspired oxygen or ventilation can cause rapid desaturation).

Immature airway and respiratory system can lead to airway obstruction during sedation or mask ventilation. In addition to this, diaphragmatic movement associated with gastric distension can also trigger significant respiratory failure. Infection, airway obstruction, hypoventilation, hypoxemia, and sepsis are among the reasons of apneic episodes [7]. Therewith, anemia may precipitate postoperative apnea and bradycardia in neonate too. Prolonged period of apnea results in hypoxia and hypercapnia. Our current knowledge shows that the risk of postoperative apnea continues in expremature infants until 60 postconceptual weeks [8]. Frequently, preterm infants are victims of respiratory failure due to the immature and sensitive respiratory structures. Many preterm infants needed increased (mechanical ventilatory support or CPAP, supplemental oxygen, etc.) respiratory support to preserve fundamental oxygenation. In hypoxic circumstances, respiratory rates of preterm and newborns decrease paradoxically.

Numerous neonatal emergency abdominal surgeries can be seen associated with respiratory system insufficiency. Respiratory variables, which are mentioned earlier, must be taken into consideration in these cases.

2.2. Cardiovascular system

The circulation of a newborn infant is a transitional characteristic. This means that, a significant decrease in pulmonary vascular resistance after birth. Patent ductus arteriosus (PDA) on the side interventricular shunts and connections are responsible from this circulation.

The fetal circulation is defined by increased PVR, decreased pulmonary blood flow, low systemic vascular resistance, and right-to-left blood flow through ductus arteriosus and foramen ovale [9, 3]. The onset of spontaneous breathing is the main factor that reduces PVR. This reduction of PVR is followed by an increase in systemic vascular resistance and left atrial pressure. Extrauterine circulation changes to a serial type of circulation as an adult.

Physiological closure of ductus arteriosus may take up to first 24 h after birth in healthy infants. However, ductus arteriosus closes anatomically after several days. Different pathological situations may cause shunting of blood via this structure. Anatomic closure of foramen ovale occurs between 3 months and 1 year of age. However, functionally closure takes place immediately. Foramen ovale may persist in 10% of the adult patients.

Reduction of pulmonary blood flow or pulmonary vasoconstriction can cause a return of the fetal circulation characteristics. This circulatory pattern is called persistent fetal circulation (PFC) or persistent pulmonary hypertension of the newborn (PPHN) [10]. Hypoxemia and acidosis can aggravate PFC. In infants with CDH, meconium aspiration and infection may be seen as PFC.

Therefore, neonatal myocardium is less compliant, and newborn's cardiac output is heart-rate dependent. The sympathetic innervation of the developing heart is decreased. In such a case, neonatal heart variable responds to vasoactive drugs.

2.3. Thermoregulation

The newborn baby has a high ratio surface area to body weight and a thin layer of subcutaneous fat tissue. Therefore, they are prone to lose heat more than older children and adults. Heat loss in newborn occurs with four different mechanisms, including evaporation, convection, conduction, and radiation.

Nonshivering thermogenesis is a primary mechanism in heat loss and regulated by brown fat [11]. Brown fat is a located adipose tissue settled in the posterior neck along the interscapular and vertebral areas.

For the reason mentioned earlier, severe temperature changes can be seen in the perioperative period. Hypothermia may trigger myocardial depression, acidosis, and delayed recovery from anesthesia. Maximal precautions should be taken to prevent hypothermia in perioperative period. Applications, which required to be done to prevent heat loss, are listed below.

- Keep the ambient temperature in neutral condition.
- Humidify and warm inspired anesthetic gases.
- Use the heated blanket, radiant warmer, and transport the neonate in a heated incubator.
- Warm blood and intravenous solutions.
- Use heating solution for cleansing the skin.

3. General principles of anesthesia in neonate

Anesthetic management of neonates that require emergency surgery is challenging and may cause serious problems to the anesthesiologist. The identification of patients at high risk for procedure-related morbidity and mortality should be a basic preventive effort. The practice of a safe anesthesia and perioperative management in such patients depends on a clear understanding of the anatomical, physiological, and hemodynamic differences and variables.

Our knowledge about pain perception in newborns has changed in recent years. Unlike the historical information, premature and term infants can feel pain from painful procedures. In recent literatures and studies, it is shown that preterm and term infants have a perception of pain, and these infants give physiological responses (such as autonomic, endocrine, and metabolic) to painful stimuli [12]. These stimulus and stress can increase pulmonary vascular resistance ergo, increase shunting through the foramen ovale, and ductus arteriosus. This phenomenon may result in hypoxemia.

Because of this, a detailed anesthesia plan should be developed for safe patient care, effective pain control, and outcome in perioperative period.

3.1. Effects of anesthetic agents

The effects of anesthetic agents vary with physical growth and changes, organ maturation, development, and coexisting disease in pediatric patient population. Inhalation anesthesia is the commonly used anesthetic technique in children. In infants, minimal alveolar concentration (MAC) is an estimate of anesthetic requirements and changes with age [8, 11]. Infants up to 6 months of age require higher MAC value than older neonates [8]. Volatile anesthetics cause dose-dependent cardiac and respiratory depressant effect in neonates. These effects can cause bradycardia, hypotension, and postoperative apnea. This hypotensive effect is more likely in preterm and term neonates than older children, especially in the induction period.

In contrast, an opioid agent causes fewer hemodynamic changes, but it should be noted that increase the risk of postoperative apnea in preterm and term neonates [2].

In the last 15 years, effects of general anesthetic agents on brain development have made a great progress. The recent animal studies have demonstrated that general anesthetics (especially these acting through the N-methyl-D-aspartate (NMDA) and Gama aminobutyric acid (GABA) receptors) can be responsible from neuronal cell death and deterioration of brain development especially immature brain [13]. It is reported that this effect is to be related to drug dosages and exposure time. Many factors affect brain maturation apart from anesthesia. Dinardo et al. emphasized that neuroanatomic abnormalities preexist in neonatal patients with complex congenital cardiac pathologies. The retardation of brain maturation has been observed in these patients [14]. Long-term neurobehavioral effects of sedative and anesthetic agents should be supported by long-term human studies.

3.2. Monitoring

Basic monitorization should include heart rate-electrocardiograph, pulse oximetry, blood pressure, and temperature in neonates. Two oxygen saturation probes must be plugged (preductal and postductal probes). This approach is intended to evaluate possible PDA-mediated shunt development. Invasive arterial blood pressure and central venous pressure can be monitored in special circumstances such as expected ventilation-perfusion and hemodynamic changes and acid-base imbalance.

Precordial-esophageal stethoscope is a very useful method in neonatal monitoring. With this method, changes in heart rate and respiratory parameters can be identified in the early phase. Although end-tidal carbon monoxide monitorization is a routine application, increase in dead space in the breathing system can cause false and inaccurate measurement in infants.

4. Anesthetic management of special neonatal surgical emergencies

4.1. Congenital diaphragmatic hernia

CDH is one of the complex and compelling anomalies in the neonatal period. CDH occurs in about 1:2400 and 1:3000 live births [8, 15]. Incomplete formation of the diaphragm and the inability of the intestines to return to the abdominal cavity result in CDH. Posterolateral foramen originated hernia (foramen of Bochdalek) constitutes 90% of the cases. In patients with CDH because of the displacement of the abdominal contents until the mediastinum, pulmonary hypoplasia (unilateral or bilateral) and possible mediastinal shift are serious problems. Less than 15% of the remaining lung volume for gas exchange indicates a poor prognosis.

Clinical presentation of CDH includes a scaphoid abdomen, increased anteroposterior diameter of the chest, bowel sounds during chest auscultation, and respiratory distress in variable degrees. Newborn babies with CDH have a 25–30% incidence of cardiac anomalies [11, 15]. Often, gastrointestinal malformations associated with skeletal abnormalities are also possible.

In radiological imaging of the chest, bowel loops in the thoracic cavity and mediastinal shift (due to compression of the lungs) are observed. Therewithal, diagnosis can be made through ultrasongraphy in utero, but this diagnosis should be confirmed in the postpartum period.

4.1.1. Preoperative evaluation

In recent years, one of the strongly highlighted issues in CDH is the timing of surgery. There is considerable argument about this topic. Current approaches, after corrective surgery, are intended to provide cardiopulmonary stabilization. CDH study group reported that only one-third of the patients underwent surgical correction in the first 24 h of life in the mid-1990s. Nowadays, the number of patients who underwent surgery within the 24 h is less than 5% [15, 16]. Because of this, it is recommended that surgical repair should be postponed until after initial resuscitation provides preoperative stabilization.

4.1.2. Preoperative ventilation strategies

The main point in the protective efforts for patients with CDH is minimizing the physiologic instability associated with pulmonary hypoplasia and pulmonary hypertension in the postnatal period. Developing ventilator strategies have played an important role in terms of reducing mortality in the last 20 years.

After delivery (in a neonate who is diagnosed during the intrauterine period) immediate endotracheal intubation (to abstain from positive pressure ventilation and pulmonary barotrauma), ventilation with small tidal volumes, and increased respiratory rates (especially in the presence of pulmonary hypoplasia) are important initial ventilatory maneuvers [8, 15, 16]. Nasogastric tube assists in decompression of gas content of the bowel and protects the lung volume.

Inflating pressures must be kept below 30 cm H_2O with a continuous monitoring of airway pressure [2]. Pulmonary barotrauma may result in serious complications such as pneumothorax, air embolism, pneumomediatinum, and soft tissue emphysema.

In the past years, perioperative management of these patients was intended to maintain adequate oxygenation and prevention of pulmonary hypertension. As hypoxemia and hypercarbia may increase pulmonary vascular pressure, hyperventilation (to lower PCO_2) of high oxygen levels was used. However, to reduce the risk of barotrauma and high mortality incidence, today with a gentle approach, permissive hypercapnia and lower percentage of oxygen are preferred [2, 15].

On this basis, the general approach in preoperative period should include reduction of pulmonary vascular resistance, recovery of pulmonary compliance, minimal ventilatory support, and regression of radiological changes.

4.1.3. *Different presurgical therapy modalities*

4.1.3.1. *Extracorporeal membrane oxygenation*

Some neonates show rapid clinical improvement, if surgery is performed within 48 h. However, some patients may require hemodynamic, respiratory, and medical supportive therapy before definitive surgery. Extracorporeal membrane oxygenation (ECMO) is one of these treatment procedures.

The first reports about ECMO in neonates with CDH were declared in the late 1970s [17]. Oxygenation index (OI)>40, $PaCO_2$ consistently >12, and A-a gradient consistently >600 mmHg were accepted indications for initiation of ECMO in the past [18]. However, nowadays, the indications for ECMO use can be summarized as unresponsiveness to treatment. Currently, more than 30% of CDH neonates are now being managed with ECMO, and it is frequently used in patients with severe reduction of pulmonary volume before surgery [2, 19].

Nonetheless, ECMO should not be used in the presence of different serious clinical cases such as intracranial hemorrhage > Grade I, presence of accompanied congenital anomalies, fatal chromosomal abnormalities, and gestational age <34 weeks [17].

Summarization—ECMO should be considered only on those infants who cannot be treated with conventional medical therapy. So ECMO is used as an additional therapy for patients who have resistant hypoxemia despite inotropic and ventilatory support.

4.1.3.2. *Ex utero intrapartum treatment (EXIT) procedure*

EXIT is an intrauterine treatment procedure in some cases of CDH. In this procedure, after fetal head removal from the uterus, fetus is intubated for assessing oxygenation or connected to the ECMO prior to umbilical cord clamping. In literature, some cases have been reported where fetal gas exchange is supported by ex utero placental circulation for over 60 minutes [2].

4.1.4. *Surgical approach and intraoperative consideration*

In the conventional approach, diaphragmatic defect is repaired via a thoracotomy incision on the ipsilateral side of the hernia. Thoracic approach is preferred in some cases. During the operation, diaphragmatic defect is repaired depending on the size of the defect. Small defects were closed primarily in which large patch graft may be required. After the closure of abdominal viscera, intraabdominal pressure may increase excessively. This clinical situation can worsen respiratory insufficiency and higher ventilation pressure should be required in the intraoperative and postoperative period. But pulmonary barotaruma should be avoided in this period.

4.1.5. Postoperative period

Severity of pulmonary hypoplasia and hypertension is an important factor that affects overall survival. Several factors affect pulmonary compliance after emergency surgery. These factors (such as increased intraabdominal pressure, lung hypoplasia, and postoperative painful stimulus) frequently cause rapid decrease in compliance. Opioids can reduce the stress response and catecholamine release in response to painful stimuli. In addition, opioids provide effective pain control so decrease the pulmonary vasoconstrictor responses to painful stimuli in neonatal intensive care unit (NICU) [2, 16].

4.2. Abdominal wall defect

4.2.1. Gastroschisis and omphalocele

Gastroschisis and omphalocele are characterized by congenital defect in the abdominal wall and herniation or evisceration of abdominal viscera [2, 20, 21]. The incidence of these defects is 1:3000 to 10000 live births [2].

Gastroschisis is defined by the absence of a division in the right abdominal wall if omphalocele is a periumbilical defect of the abdominal wall and a majority in male neonate [2]. Current knowledge supports the fact that omphalocele and gastroschisis arise from separate embryologic processes. Herniation of abdominal contents overlaps with a translucent lamina of peritoneum. The characteristic of the lesion is amniotic membrane. In addition, the intestines, spleen, and liver may be located in a large defect. Both clinical cases should require emergency surgical approach due to rapid and substantial heat and fluid losses by extra abdominal organs (especially bowels). Some congenital anomalies are often associated with omphalocele such as trisomies, congenital cardiac anomalies (e.g., Fallot tetralogy), Bechwith-Wiedemann syndrome, malrotation of the intestine, chromosomal anomalies, and meningocele [21, 2]. Prematurity is an important factor that increases mortality in these patients.

4.2.2. Preoperative period

Although each of the lesions is a different etiology, approaches are similar for both the pathologies. The preoperative fundamental approach to abdominal wall defects primarily includes adequate fluid resuscitation to prevent heat loss and treatment of infection and sepsis to avoid direct trauma to the eviscerated organs [11]. In both the cases for the prevention, the defect (especially large defect) is covered with sterile wet dressing [22].

Dense fluid replacement therapy is required and is vital for these patients. The stomach should be decompressed with a nasogastric tube. This process is intended to reduce regurgitation, aspiration, and bowel distention. Systemic antibiotics should be started primarily. Intense protein loss and translocation of fluid into third space can be seen in ruptured cases. Oncotic pressure is also decreased. Arterial blood gas analysis should be performed.

4.2.3. Intraoperative management

Major issues that we need to pay attention in preoperative approach are also important in the intraoperative period. The maintenance of body temperature and adequate fluid resuscitation should be noted. Because of this, adequate intravenous access must be ensured and invasive monitoring is necessary if an associated cardiac defect is present.

Surgical intervention is required to reduce the bowel back into the abdominal cavity and repair the abdominal wall defect. Different surgical techniques (such as primary closure in the operating room or bedside, placement of a prefabricated silastic silos or fashioning of a hand-sewn silo) are applicable [23]. Silo method is a transition repair procedure. Some infants may remain intubated until final closure in the NICU setting. Nowadays, the sutureless umbilical closure has become a widely accepted technique [24]. In the renewed procedure, herniated viscera are reduced into the abdomen. Umbilical cord is used to pack the abdominal wall defect. This technique may be implemented at the bedside in the neonatal intensive care unit. Nevertheless, in patients with larger defect, surgery should be performed in the operating room. Anesthetic management consists of endotracheal intubation in the awakened patients with gastric decompression after preoxygenation. Anesthesia is maintained with inhalational anesthetics and controlled ventilation. Muscle relaxants may be used to provide optimal surgical circumstances for closure of the defect.

It must be kept in mind that if abdominal defects are closed too tightly, abdominal pressure can increase because of underdeveloped abdominal cavity. This situation can lead to respiratory failure, diminish visceral organ and lower extremity perfusion, and decrease venous return due to caval compression [8]. In this situation, postoperative ventilatory support may be necessary. In patients with associated anomalies, close monitoring (especially airway pressure and central venous pressure) is vital and invasive blood pressure monitorization and arterial blood gas analysis may be useful and observational hemodynamic parameters provide optimal oxygenation and fluid therapy. Respiratory parameters should be monitored closely after surgery. Postoperative mechanical ventilatory support is recommended during 24–48 h in NICU. Prolonged ileus after surgery may cause parenteral nutrition in a longer period.

4.3. Necrotizing enterocolitis

Necrotizing enterocolitis (NEC) is one of the important cause of morbidity and mortality that particularly affects premature infants under 36 weeks of gestational age (usually premature infants fewer than 32 weeks) [2, 16, 21]. The causes of NEC are still unclear. However, the etiology of NEC is considered multifactorial. Prematurity is a definite risk factor mainly affecting premature infants fewer than 32 weeks' gestation and body weight is less than 1500 gr. In addition, hypoxemia, enteral feedings (especially hyperosmolar solutions), cyanotic heart disease, and PDA have been suggested as risk factors. Although the etiology is different, the result is increased mucosal permeability, intestinal ischemia, and sepsis.

Clinical features of these patients are characterized by abdominal distention, retained gastric secretion, bloody stool, and bile-stained aspirates [2, 25]. In some cases, irritability, lethargia, apnea, and temperature instability may accompany this situation. Hypovolemic shock can be seen in cases with generalized peritonitis. A hemorrhagic diathesis with thrombocytopenia may emerge in septic infants. Many of these infants who have developing respiratory insufficiency and hyaline membrane syndrome require intubation and mechanical ventilation support.

It is important to know the risk factors, and early diagnosis and initial treatment in these patients are also necessary. Some cases including less severe ones can be treated with broad-spectrum antibiotics, intravenous fluids, and nasogastric decompression. However, acute phase of NEC required emergency surgery, and pneumoperitoneum is an absolute indication [25, 26]. Positive paracentesis, constant abdominal mass, fixed dilated intestinal loop, and progressive metabolic acidosis are among relative surgical indications [2, 16, 21].

4.3.1. Intraoperative management

Intraoperative approach in patients with NEC should contain close monitoring of invasive arterial and central venous pressure, blood gas, and metabolic analysis. Blood products (such as red blood cells, fresh frozen plasma, and platelets) may be required in infants with coagulaopathies in the early period. In addition, severe hypovolemia is a significant problem in these infants and requires intensive treatment with crystalloid and colloid solutions.

Potent inhalational anesthetics can aggravate a hypovolemic situation. Because of this, frequently inhalational anesthetics are utilized in low concentration to supplement opioids. High-dose opioid (especially fentanyl) is a safe and viable option for balanced anesthesia [8]. Nitrous oxide should not be used. Because of the risk of premature retinopathy, inspired oxygen concentration should be calibrated to keep between an arterial oxygen saturation of 85–90% [16].

Neuromuscular blockers may be used to facilitate surgical intervention. Hemodynamic collapse is often in these newborns. In this regard, despite fluid resuscitation in patients who are not provided adequate perfusion, inotropic agents are often necessary to protect cardiovascular stability. Glucose intolerance is a significant problem particularly in septic patients. Intermittently, arterial blood gas analysis and glucose measurement is an important measurement parameter.

4.3.2. Postoperative consideration

These infants often require postoperative mechanical ventilatory and cardiovascular support. Parenteral nutrition is necessary after sepsis is controlled and metabolic stability is maintained [20].

4.4. Esophageal malformations

4.4.1. Esophageal atresia, tracheoesophageal fistula

Esophageal atresia is the most common esophageal malformation. The incidence reported is at 1 in 2500–3000 live births [27].

Esophageal malformations can manifest in five different forms according to localization of atresia and presence of fistula. The most common defect (80–90%) consists of a blind, upper esophageal pouch with distal tracheoesophageal fistula.

Severe cardiovascular anomalies (such as ventricular septal defect, coarctation of aorta, and Tetralogy of Fallot,) can be associated with esophageal atresia. This anomaly can also be a part of a syndrome known as VATER [vertebra (V) anal (A), tracheoesophageal (TE), renal (R)] or VATER syndrome associated cardiac (C) and limb (L) anomalies called VACTERL syndrome [8, 27]. These associated anomalies worsen the prognosis.

Prenatal diagnosis can be made with the ultrasound. Inability to swallow, choking attacks, aspiration, and abdominal distention should be preoccupying esophageal atresia in the early postnatal period. The disability of the nasogastric tube to pass through the atretic esophagus passage is also seen in the clinical examination.

Definitive diagnosis is made by contrast radiological examination. Pulmonary aspiration, other causes of abdominal distention, and prematurity-dependent problems should be considered in differential diagnosis. Preoperative echocardiography must be performed owing to the associated congenital cardiac anomalies. Concomitant cardiac anomalies and birth weight are among the factors affecting mortality in patients with Tracheoesophageal Fistula (TEF)/EA.

4.4.2. Anesthetic management

The operation of TEF is acceptable and urgent, but not immediate, and the time of surgery is determined by the general condition of the infant. Considering the general condition of the patients, surgical approach can be planned—primary closure of the fistula and anastomosis, gastrostomy before or after definitive surgery, or a delayed primary closure [28]. In patients, who provide clinical improvement, surgery can be carried out within 24–72 h [11]. Antibiotic therapy should be initiated immediately in infants with pulmonary infection. In these cases, surgery may be delayed as much as clinically stability. Despite the intensive, care, support, and antibiotic therapy, if there is continuous clinical worsening and respiratory insufficiency, immediate surgery may be necessary.

However, if the scheduled surgery is delayed, usually fistula is closed, and gastrostomy is performed. Gastrostomy is used to decompress the stomach and decrease regurgitation into the lungs. In addition, gastrostomy provides nutritional support in cases in which definitive surgery is delayed. This process can take 3–6 months.

The basic preoperative anesthetic management in patients undergoing surgical approach includes the following:

- Degree of neonatal age (especially prematurity) and associated congenital anomalies
- Interruption of feeding and intermittent aspiration of the upper esophageal pouch
- Prevent excessive gastric distention due to air intake into the stomach through the fistula

- Evaluation of aspiration pneumonia, if necessary, antibiotic therapy to treat pulmonary infection

Before management of anesthesia, aspiration catheter may be useful to drain secretions in the esophagus. In anesthesia, induction should be administered carefully to prevent abdominal distention and pulmonary aspiration. In general, intubation is performed in awake conditions. Sedation can be administered with titrated dose of fentanyl (0.5–1 $\mu g\ kg^{-1}$) and 25–50 $\mu g\ kg^{-1}$ midazolam [8]. Also deep inhalational anesthesia to induction may be preferable to endotracheal intubation. In this period, maintenance of spontaneous breathing should be noted. Muscle relaxant may be an addition after the ligation of fistula.

The placement of the endotracheal tube (ETT) is important. ETT tip must be above the carina, but it must be placed below the fistula. It may not be easy to find the correct tube localization. Generally, tube is advanced through the right mainstem bronchus and then pulled back slightly until breath sounds are heard bilaterally. Tube localization can be confirmed by flexible fiberoptic bronchoscope [29]. Even with initial optimal position of the ETT, in some patients, ventilation through the fistula still occurs, and this is particularly seen in patients who require high peak airway pressure. In these cases, the use of low inspiratory pressure will prevent gastric distention until the ligation of the fistula.

In appropriate cases, a primary repair can be performed, the fistula is ligated, and esophagus is primary anastomosed. Intraoperatively, retraction of the lung may be required to provide proper exposure intraoperatively. In this period, deterioration of oxygenation is a common problem due to collapsed lung experience by an anesthesiologist. Intermittent ventilation of collapsed lung and close cooperation of surgical team may improve oxygenation.

In addition, precordial stethoscope should be a part of an intraoperative monitorization during repair of the TEF. Precordial stethoscope is placed in the left axilla to assess the adequacy of ventilation in the dependent lung. In infants with associated anomalies such as congenital cardiac defect or hemodynamic instability, invasive arterial monitoring should be performed.

Two oxygen saturation probes may be helpful to evaluate pre- and postductal oxygen saturation and shunt fraction via patent ductus arteriosus.

4.4.3. Postoperative approach

In patients with TEF, significant pathological finding is a reduced amount of tracheal cartilage. Tracheomalacia or defective tracheal wall can cause airway collapse. Therefore, most patients require postoperative ventilatory support in early postoperative period (at least 24–48 h) in NICU. This period may take up 5–7 days in infants who have long gap anastomosis [8, 16, 29]. Intermittent arterial blood gas analysis and chest radiographs will be useful in the postoperative follow-up period.

Opioid infusion is effective in the treatment of postoperative pain and sedation in this period.

Anastomotic leak and strictures are main complications in early postoperative period. Structural and functional abnormalities (such as gastroesophageal reflux and chronic pulmonary disease) are considerable problems that may be encountered in the long-term period [2, 30].

Therefore, it should be noted that EA or TEF is not a small anatomic problem that completely ameliorates by surgical approach.

5. A Special highlight for pediatric spinal anesthesia

In the last 30 decades, pediatric spinal anesthesia has become one of the most attractive and popular topics in anesthesia practice with the increase of our knowledge and experience on this issue. Despite the growing interest, spinal anesthesia requires technical expertise, and it is not still performed in many centers. Notwithstanding, general anesthesia is a standard technique for many pediatric anesthetist.

Spinal anesthesia has become a considerable anesthetic technique for reducing the risk of postoperative apnea in premature and ex-premature infants [31]. Unsupplemented spinal anesthesia may be used in lower abdominal surgery (such as necrotizing enterocolitis, pyloromyotomi, omphalocele, and gastroschisis) in neonatal age group. Abajian et al. in 1984 reported the use of spinal anesthesia in high-risk ex-premature infants and considered regional anesthesia by spinal approach to be safe and effective in these patients [32].

At the same time, spinal anesthesia is characterized by remarkable hemodynamic stability in neonate and infant patients. In reference [33] this physiological characteristic means that minimum or no cardiodepressant effect and is important especially in the neonatal period. Because neonatal heart just after birth is more immature than adult heart and have a lower velocity of contraction and a minimize length-tension correlation.

In infants with limited pulmonary perfusion, it is important to maintain systemic vascular resistance and control of PVR and pulmonary blood flow. Some of these patients require immediate surgical intervention. In these patients, spinal block decreases undesirable adverse effects related to the sympathetic system activity.

Surgical trauma and pain cause a hormonal stress response that is directly related to the severity and urgency of surgery. Spinal anesthesia is an effective pain control technique. Thus, hormonal stress response and catecholamine release reduces in intraoperative and postoperative period [31, 34].

In the previous studies, it has been suggested that when compared with general anesthesia, spinal anesthesia is associated with fewer cardiovascular and respiratory complications, and there is less need for postoperative mechanical ventilation and a shorter hospital stay [35].

Because of these factors, it has to be kept in mind that spinal anesthesia seems reliable and a safe alternative technique in selected cases especially for specific lower abdominal surgery.

6. Summary

Preterm and term neonates may need various surgical interventions, but unfortunately, many of them are urgent. Newborn period is a challenging period for the anesthesiologist. This difficulty is caused by many factors related to neonatal population such as immaturity of physiological processes, organs, and systems, and pathophysiological instability caused by the underlying comorbidities and associated congenital anomalies. For these reasons, anesthesia-associated morbidity and mortality is greater in this group than in older infants and children. A cautious approach to all aspects of perioperative care is vital to minimize the possible side effects. The basics of safe anesthetic management in preterm and term neonates are summarized in this chapter, based on emergency abdominal surgery.

Author details

Esra Caliskan

Address all correspondence to: duru5654@gmail.com

Department of Anesthesiology and Reanimation, Baskent University, Faculty of Medicine, Ankara, Turkey

References

[1] Partridge EA, Flake AW. Maternal-fetal surgery for structural malformations. Best Pract Res Clin Obstet Gynaecol. 2012; 26:669–682. DOI: 10.1016/j.bpobgyn.2012.03.003.

[2] Brusseau R, McCann ME. Anaesthesia for urgent and emergency surgery. Early Hum Dev 2010; 86:703–714. DOI: 10.1016/j.earlhumdev.2010.08.008.

[3] Motoyoma EK, Finder JD. Respiratory physiology in Infants and Children. In: Davis PJ, Cladis FP, Motoyoma EK editors. Smith's Anesthesia for Infants and Children. 8th ed. Philadelphia: Elsevier; 2011. Pp. 23–41. ISBN: 978-0-323-06612-9. ch3.

[4] Joshi S, Kotecha S. Lung growth and development. Early Hum Dev 2007; 83:789–794. DOI: 10.1016/j.earlhumdev.2007.09.007.

[5] Finnemore A, Groves A. Physiology of the fetal and transitional circulation. Semin Fetal Neonatal Med 2015; 20:210–216. DOI: 10.1016/j.siny.2015.04.003.

[6] Souza DD, McDaniel GM, Baum VC. Cardiovascular physiology. In: Davis PJ, Cladis FP, Motoyoma EK editors. Smith's Anesthesia for Infants and Children. 8th ed. Philadelphia: Elsevier; 2011. Pp. 81–115. ISBN: 978-0-323-06612-9. ch4.

[7] Sale SM. Neonatal apnoea. Best Pract Res Clin Anaesthesiol 2010; 24:323–336. DOI: 10.1016/j.bpa.2010.04.002.

[8] Cote CJ. Pediatric anetshesia. In: Miller RD, editor. Miller's Anesthesia. 7th ed. Philadelphia: Churchill Livingstone; 2010. Pp. 2559–2597. ISBN: 978-0-443-06959-8.ch.

[9] Hines MH. Neonatal cardiovascular physiology. Semin Pediatr Surg 2013; 22:174–178. DOI: 10.1053/j.sempedsurg.2013.10.004.

[10] Jain A, McNamara PJ. Persistent pulmonary hypertension of the newborn: advances in diagnosis and treatment. Semin Fetal Neonat Med 2015; 20: 262–271. DOI: 10.1016/j.siny.2015.03.001

[11] Gregory GA, Brett C. Neonatology for anesthesiologist. In: Davis PJ, Cladis FP, Motoyoma EK Editors. Smith's Anesthesia for Infants and Children. 8th ed. Philadelphia: Elsevier; 2011, pp. 513–553. ISBN: 978-0-323-06612-9. ch17.

[12] Anand KJS. Pharmacological approaches to the management of pain in the neonatal intensive care unit. J Perinatol 2007; 27:S4–S111. DOI: 10.1038/sj.jp.7211712.

[13] Sun L. Early childhood general anesthesia exposure and neurocognitive development. Br J Anaesth 2010; 105: i61–i68. DOI: 10.1093/bja/aeq302.

[14] DiNardo JA. Should what we know about neurobehavioral development, complex congenital heart disease, and brain maturation affect the timing of corrective cardiac surgery? Paediatr Anaesth. 2011; 21: 781–6. DOI: 10.1111/j.1460-9592.2010.03429.

[15] Lally KP. Congenital diapragmatic hernia—the past 25(or so) years. J Pediat Surg 2016. Available from http://dx.doi.org/10.1016/j.jpedsurg2016.02.005.

[16] Brett C, Davis PJ. Anesthesia for general surgery in the neonate. In: Davis PJ, Cladis FP, Motoyoma EK editors. Smith's Anesthesia for Infants and Children. 8th ed. Philadelphia: Elsevier; 2011; pp. 554–588. ISBN: 978-0-323-06612-9. ch18.

[17] Harting MT, Lally KP. Surgical management of neonates with congenital diapragmatic hernia. Semin Ped Surg 2007; 16:109–114. DOI: 10.1053/j.sempedsurg.2007.01.007.

[18] Hedrick HL. Evaluation and management of congenital diapragmatic hernia. Pediatr Case Rev 2001; 1:25–36. DOI: 10.1097/00132584-200110000-00004.

[19] Tiruvoipati R, Vinogradova Y, Faulkner G, Sosnowski AW, Firmin RK,Peek GJ. Predictors of outcome in patients with congenital diapragmatic hernia requiring extracorporeal membrane oxygenation. J Pediatr Surg 2007; 42:98–104. DOI: 10. 1016/j.jpedsurg.2007.03.031

[20] Chesley PM, Letbetter DJ, Meehan JJ, Oron AP, Javid PJ. Contemporary trends in the use of primary repair for gastroschisis in surgical infants. Am J Surg 2015; 209: 901–906. DOI: 10.1016/j.amjsurg.2015.01.012.

[21] Dierdorf SF, Krishna G. Anesthetic Management of Neonatal Surgical Emergencies. Anesth Analg 1981; 60: 204–214. ISSN: 0003-2999.

[22] Mann L, Ferguson-Smith MA, Desai M, Gibson AA, Raine PA. Prenatal assessment of anterior abdominal wall defects and their prognosis. Prenat Diagn 1984; 4: 427–435. DOI: 10.1002/pd.1970040606.

[23] Aldrink HJ, Caniano DA, Nwomeh BC. Variability in gastroschisis management: a survey of North American pediatric surgery training programs. J Surg Res 2012; 176:159–163. DOI: 10.1016/j.jss.2011.05.012.

[24] Riboh J, Abrajano C, Garber K, et al. Outcome of sutureless gastroschisis closure. J Pediatr Surg 2009; 44: 1947–1951. DOI: 10.1016/j.jpedsurg.2009.03.027.

[25] Bayley G. Special considerations in the premature and ex-premature infant. Anaesth Intensive Care Med 2014; 15: 107–110. DOI: 10.1016/j.mpaic.2008.01.007.

[26] Pierro A. The surgical management of necrotising enterocolitis. Early Hum Dev 2005; 81(1): 79–85. DOI: 10.1016/j.earlhumdev.2004.10.018.

[27] Natasha Broemling N, Campbell F. Anesthetic management of congenital tracheoesophageal fistula. Pediatr Anesth 2011; 21: 1092–1099. DOI: 10.1111/j.1460-9592.2010.03377.

[28] Andropoulos DB, Rowe RW, Betts JM. Anaesthetic and surgical airway management during trachea-oesophagial fistula repair. Pediatr Anesth 1998; 8:313–319. DOI: 10.1046/j.1460-9592.1998.00734.

[29] Broemling N, Campbell F. Anesthetic management of congenital tracheoesophageal fistula. Pediatr Anesth 2011; 21:1092–1099. DOI: 10.1111/j.1460-9592.2010.03377.

[30] Marseglia L, Manti S, D'Angelo G, Gitto E, Salpietro C, Centorrino A et al. Gastroesophagial reflux and congenital gastrointestinal malformations. World J Gastroenterol 2015; 21: 8508–8515. DOI: 10.3748/wjg.v21.i28.8508.

[31] Bosenberg A. Benefits of regional anesthesia in children. Pediatr Anesth 2012; 22:10–18. DOI: 10.1111/j.1460-9592.2011.03691.

[32] Abajian JC, Mellish RW, Browne AF, Perkins FM, Lambert DH, Mazuzan JE Jr. Spinal anesthesia for surgery in the high-risk infant. Anesth Analg 1984; 63:359-362. ISSN: 0003-2999.

[33] Shenkman Z, Johnson VM, Zurakowski D, et al. Hemodynamic changes during spinal anesthesia in premature infants with congenital heart disease undergoing inguinal hernia correction. Pediatr Anesth 2012; 22:865–870. DOI: 10.1111/j.1460-9592.2012.03873.

[34] Wolf AR, Doyle E, Thomas E. Modifying infant stress responses to major surgery: spinal vs extradural vs opiod analgesia. Pediatr Anesth 1998; 8:305–311. DOI: 10.1046/j.1460-592.1998.00239.

[35] White MC. Approach to managing children with heart disease for noncardiac surgery. Pediatr Anesth 2011; 21:522–529. DOI: 10.1111/j.1460 j.1460-9592.2010.03416.